Synopsis of
Postmortem CT
& CT Angiography
for Death Investigation

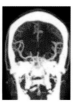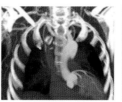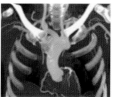

Synopsis of
Postmortem CT and CT Angiography
for Death Investigation

1st Edition Printed | August 9, 2021
1st Edition Issued | August 23, 2021

Edited by	Heon Lee and Sookyoung Lee.
Authors by	Heon Lee, Sookyoung Lee, Jang Gyu Cha, Taewha Baik, and Kyung-moo Yang
Planned by	Hyeong-seok Jo
Publisher	Ju-Yeon Chang
Editing Design by	Eun-jung Yang
Cover Design by	Jae-wook Kim
Publishing House	Koonja Publishing, Inc.

Registration No. 4-139 (June 24, 1991)
Paju Publishing Complex, 338, Hoedong-gil (474-1 Seopae-dong),
Paju-si, Gyeonggi-do, South Korea (10881)
Telephone: (031) 943-1888 Fax: (031) 955-9545
Website: www.koonja.co.kr

ISBN 979-11-5955-738-5

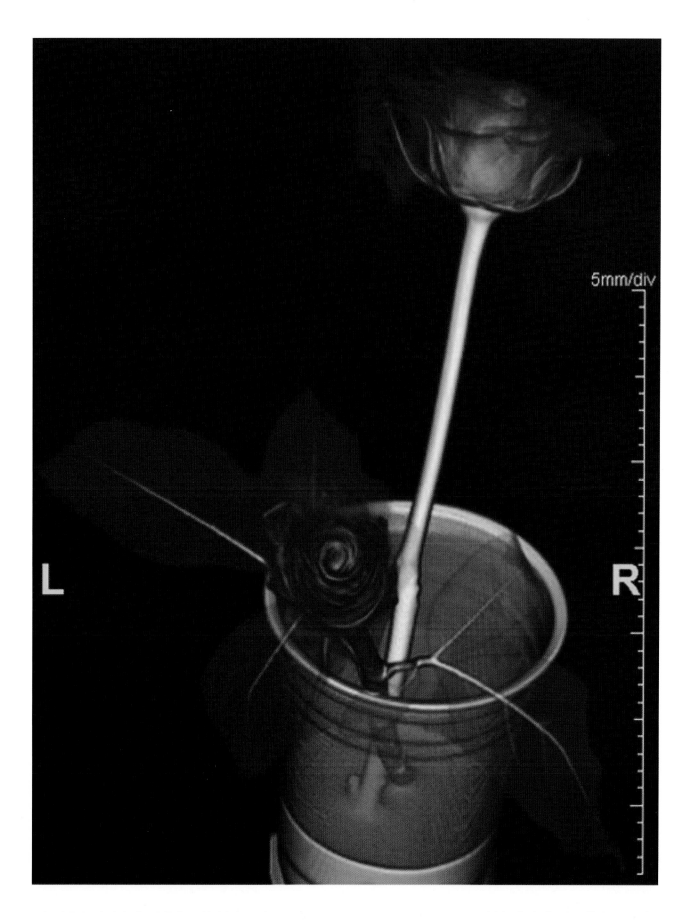

PREFACE

The idea for writing the book "**Synopsis of Postmortem CT and CT Angiography for Death Investigation**" originated from a sincere and longstanding collaboration between clinical radiologists at Soonchunhyang University Hospital Bucheon and forensic pathologists working for the National Forensic Service, Republic of Korea (NFS Korea). Over the past 10 years, they have been at the forefront of introducing and operating computed tomography (CT) systems in forensic and medicolegal death investigations in Korea. Their unique partnership helped them to implement a head-to-head comparison between imaging findings and autopsy results. This direct radiological-pathological comparison has provided excellent learning tools and opportunities for both radiologists and pathologists to address a wide variety of challenging forensic and medicolegal questions. We believe that this collaboration of expertise based on mutual understanding will continue to benefit forensic science for many years to come.

In recent years, with the introduction of modern imaging technology into the forensic field, postmortem cross-sectional imaging, particularly CT and CT angiography, has gained increasing attention in the field of death investigation worldwide. These CT techniques play roles in screening for potential pathologies, guiding subsequent autopsy dissection to the target area, and identifying lesions that are difficult or impossible to detect during conventional autopsy dissection. For clinical radiologists, it has always been essential to understand the pathological basis of disease for accurate interpretation of imaging studies in clinical settings. In addition, knowledge of normal postmortem changes in tissue and the corresponding CT findings that may produce artifacts is required for death investigations. Furthermore, to obtain the greatest benefit from these imaging techniques, pathologists are strongly recommended to have an understanding of the basic principles behind CT (i.e., how CT images are produced, reconstructed, and interpreted). This understanding is especially important when real-time assistance in CT acquisition and image interpretation from forensic radiologists is unavailable.

In preparing this book, our primary goal was to introduce clinical radiologists to emerging postmortem CT (PMCT) techniques and provide them with essential knowledge of typical postmortem body changes and perimortem artifacts to prevent misinterpretation of those findings as true pathologies. We presume that a high level of familiarity with the capabilities and limitations of PMCT and PMCT angiography (PMCTA) techniques will help radiologists to prepare for forthcoming collaboration and communication with forensic pathologists.

Our secondary goal for this book was to provide pathologists with a technical basis and interpretive fundamentals for the application of modern CT imaging to their daily routine. Accordingly, as a guide to PMCT imaging, particular focus has been placed on the pictorial depiction of representative cases that demonstrate the diagnostic aids of PMCT and PMCTA in death investigations. We have presented these cases in a few relevant images using various reconstruction techniques to condense the corresponding diagnostic information in an intuitive manner. In each case, corresponding autopsy photographs and brief forensic information were added, facilitating a comprehensive understanding of the cases for pathologists who are not familiar with PMCT imaging.

After a concise description of the historical background of forensic imaging and technical considerations of CT in part I, we address the advantages and limitations of PMCT and PMCTA in two major categories of death: traumatic (e.g., blunt trauma, sharp force injury, gunshot wounds, blast injury, strangulation, and drowning) in parts II and III, and non-traumatic (e.g., natural death and death with a medicolegal component) in part III. We provide a brief discussion of radiological and pathological findings, with particular emphasis on the diagnostic values of these techniques during death investigations. In part IV, we describe normal postmortem changes and decomposition that begin to occur immediately after death and may be misdiagnosed as true pathologies or mask the true lesions on CT images. In addition, we discuss artifacts related to CT and angiographic techniques with their remedies.

We believe that this small book will be particularly useful for forensic pathologists and clinical radiologists who expect to be involved in PMCT imaging or who have a plan to use CT for forensic purposes in their institutions, thus providing a practical and informative guide to PMCT imaging. We also hope that this book helps those interested in or involved with forensic science, regardless of their specialty, to understand better the current role and future potential of imaging in daily death investigation.

Heon Lee MD, PhD for all Authors

ACKNOWLEDGMENTS

The authors thank the Forensic Pathologists and Radiographers of the NFS Korea for their assistance in the preparation of this manuscript. Their profound knowledge and experience in the field of forensic pathology and CT technology have supported the correlation between imaging and pathology, and aided demonstration of the additional benefits of postmortem CT and angiography, which this book is aimed at describing. Our publication efforts would have been futile without their help and advice.

THE EDITORS

Heon Lee MD, PhD, earned his medical degree from Jeonbuk National University College of Medicine in Jeonju, South Korea and he is a certified radiologist by the Korean board of Radiology. After completion of one year fellowship training of cardiovascular imaging at Medical University of South Carolina in Charleston SC 2007, he served as director of the radiology department at Seoul Medical Center. He is currently a tenured professor in the department of radiology at Soonchunhyang University Hospital Bucheon and a consultant radiologist of NFS Korea. His main scientific interest is non-invasive cardiovascular imaging, especially using advanced CT and MRI techniques for the diagnosis of cardiovascular diseases and injuries for both clinical and forensic purposes. Currently, he has been involved in many research projects with NFS Korea, including the application of postmortem CT/CT angiography in death investigation and the development of automated injectors and contrast agents for postmortem use.
E-mail: acarad@naver.com

Sookyoung Lee MD, PhD, received his medical degree from Kyungbuk National University College of Medicine in Daegu, South Korea and he is a certified pathologist by the Korean society of pathology. After completing one year of forensic training in the Forensic Institute at LMU Munich University and Wayne County Medical Examiner Office in Detroit respectively, he worked as a professor of pathology at Soonchunhyang University Hospital Cheonan. He is currently a forensic pathologist in charge of CT imaging laboratory at NFS Korea. He has been deeply interested in application of postmortem CT imaging in daily forensic practice and involved in several research projects to develop dedicated postmortem contrast agents and injectors.
E-mail: heart@korea.kr

CONTRIBUTING AUTHORS

Heon Lee MD, PhD

Professor, Department of Radiology, Soonchunhyang University Hospital Bucheon, Bucheon;
Consultant Radiologist, Department of Forensic Medicine, National Forensic Service, Wonju, Republic of Korea

Sookyoung Lee MD, PhD

Forensic Pathologist, Director of Forensic Medical Examination Division,
National Forensic Service, Wonju, Republic of Korea

Jang Gyu Cha MD, PhD.

Professor, Department of Radiology, Soonchunhyang University Hospital Bucheon, Bucheon;
Consultant Radiologist, Department of Forensic Medicine, National Forensic Service, Wonju, Republic of Korea

Taewha Baik MD, PhD.

Forensic pathologist, Department of Forensic Medicine, National Forensic Service, Wonju, Republic of Korea

Kyung-moo Yang, MD, PhD.

Forensic pathologist, Director General of Department of Forensic Medicine,
National Forensic Service, Wonju, Republic of Korea

CONTENTS

Part I. **Application of CT in postmortem imaging**
– an emerging subspecialty of radiology

Part II. **Traumatic death**

Part III. **Death by asphyxiation**

Part IV. **Nontraumatic death**

Part V. **Artifacts frequently found on postmortem CT and CTA**

Application of CT in postmortem imaging
- an emerging subspecialty of radiology

"The Stone Age didn't end for lack of stone"
– Ahmed Zaki Yamani, 1930−2021

Chapter 01

Brief history of forensic imaging

The forensic use of radiography began immediately after Professor Roentgen's discovery of X-rays. Since its first successful use in a gunshot case in early 1896 to identify bullets in the victim's body[1], X-ray radiography has been used for screening of the body (Fig. 1) and is now widely applied for locating foreign materials in blast and firearm injuries, skeletal surveys in cases of child abuse, and identification in situations involving mass casualties.[2, 3]

Computed tomography (CT) imaging was first introduced in a death investigation in 1983 to demonstrate fatal air embolism in diving-related deaths.[4] Subsequently, advances in CT technology, (i.e., multi-detector technology and image reconstruction techniques) have enabled whole-body scanning and the display of two-dimensional (2D) and three-dimensional (3D) images involving various image planes. Postmortem CT (PMCT) examinations have been incorporated into routine forensic practice in many forensic institutions worldwide, mostly for the pre-autopsy screening of potential causes of death

and guidance of autopsy confirmation as an adjunct to autopsy dissection.[5-7] Because of its low tissue contrast, PMCT alone is unsuitable for evaluating the vascular structure, particularly in cases of death by natural causes (e.g., coronary artery disease). To address this concern, contrast infusion, as performed in clinical CT studies, has also been applied during death investigations by injecting iodinated contrast agents mixed with large amounts of volume expanders specifically designed for postmortem purposes.[8, 9] Reflecting postmortem vascular changes (i.e., the absence of circulation and collapse of the vessels)[10], PMCT angiography (PMCTA) involves separate injections of those contrast mixtures into arteries and veins, using various types of injection pumps to expand the collapsed vascular lumen. PMCTA has become a promising tool for objective and reproducible inspection of the vascular system in a minimally invasive manner.[5, 7-9]

Since an early report regarding the potential for magnetic resonance (MR) imaging as a pre-autopsy

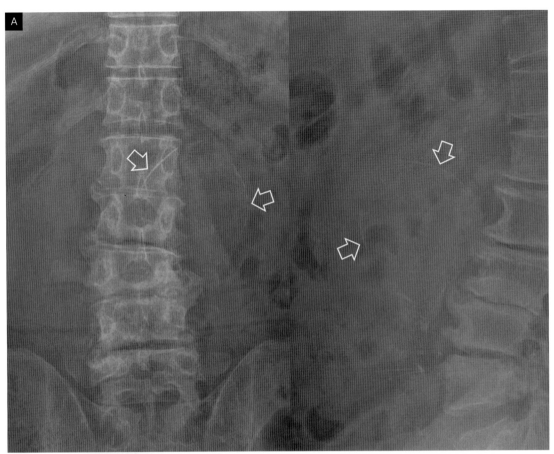

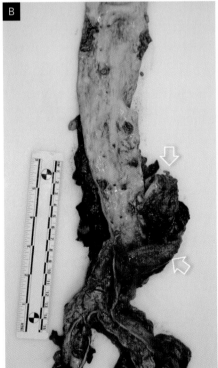

Figure 1. A 63-year-old male found dead at his home. (A) Anteroposterior and lateral views of plain abdominal radiographs show eggshell-like calcification (arrows) in the potential position of the abdominal aorta, which suggest abnormal dilatation of a calcified aortic wall (e.g., abdominal aortic aneurysm). (B) Autopsy photograph reveals abdominal aortic aneurysm (arrows) and its rupture as the cause of death.

imaging tool in death investigation in 1990[11], the excellent soft tissue contrast of MR imaging and its ability to demonstrate fluid collection have aided in the early diagnosis of various pathologies (e.g., soft tissue edema, internal hemorrhage, bone bruise, fluid collections in body spaces, and early myocardial injury due to ischemia).[12-14] Despite early favorable reports, the use of MR imaging in the postmortem setting has been limited by practical concerns such as the cost and availability of MR scanners, as well as the technical complexity, long scan time, and MR artifacts related to postmortem body changes (i.e., cessation of circulation, reduction of body temperature, and production of putrefactive gas).[6, 10, 15]

In Korea, a dedicated CT scanner for postmortem use was installed in the National Forensic Service (NFS) Seoul institute on June 18, 2013. The first postmortem CT angiography examination was performed on August 6, 2014. Subsequently, two more CT systems have been used in the NFS Wonju headquarter and NFS Pusan institute as pre-autopsy imaging tools for death investigations, and more than 4,000 PMCT examinations have been performed nationwide every year.

References

1 Eckert WG, Garland N. The history of the forensic applications in radiology. The American journal of forensic medicine and pathology. 1984;5(1):53-6. doi: 10.1097/00000433-198403000-00010.

2 Singleton AC. The roentgenological identification of victims of the "Noronic" disaster. The American journal of roentgenology and radium therapy. 1951;66(3):375-84.

3 Viner MD. The Use of Radiology in Mass Fatality Events. In: Adams BJ, Byrd JE, editors. Recovery, Analysis, and Identification of Commingled Human Remains. Totowa, NJ: Humana Press; 2008. p. 145-84.

4 Krantz P, Holtås S. Postmortem computed tomography in a diving fatality. Journal of computer assisted tomography. 1983;7(1):132-4. doi: 10.1097/00004728-198302000-00024.

5 Ross SG, Bolliger SA, Ampanozi G, Oesterhelweg L, Thali MJ, Flach PM. Postmortem CT angiography: capabilities and limitations in traumatic and natural causes of death. Radiographics: a review publication of the Radiological Society of North America, Inc. 2014; 34(3):830-46. doi: 10.1148/rg.343115169.

6 Grabherr S, Egger C, Vilarino R, Campana L, Jotterand M, Dedouit F. Modern post-mortem imaging: an update on recent developments. Forensic sciences research. 2017;2(2):52-64. doi: 10.1080/20961790. 2017.1330738.

7 Lee H, Lee S, Cha JG, Baek T, Yang KM. Postmortem Computed Tomography and Computed Tomography Angiography: Cardiothoracic Imaging Applications in Forensic Medicine. Journal of thoracic imaging. 2019;34(5):286-98. doi: 10.1097/rti.0000000000000398.

8 Ross S, Spendlove D, Bolliger S, Christe A, Oesterhelweg L, Grabherr S, et al. Postmortem whole-body CT angiography: evaluation of two contrast media solutions. AJR American journal of roentgenology. 2008;190(5):1380-9. doi: 10.2214/ajr.07.3082.

9 Grabherr S, Grimm J, Dominguez A, Vanhaebost J, Mangin P. Advances in post-mortem CT-angiography. The British journal of radiology. 2014;87(1036):20130488. doi: 10.1259/bjr.20130488.

10 Grabherr S, Grimm J, Baumann P, Mangin P. Application of contrast media in post-mortem imaging (CT and MRI). La Radiologia medica. 2015;120(9):824-34. doi: 10.1007/s11547-015-0532-2.

11 Ros PR, Li KC, Vo P, Baer H, Staab EV. Preautopsy magnetic resonance imaging: initial experience. Magnetic resonance imaging. 1990;8(3):303-8. doi: 10.1016/0730-725x(90)90103-9.

12 Ruder TD, Ebert LC, Khattab AA, Rieben R, Thali MJ, Kamat P. Edema is a sign of early acute myocardial infarction on postmortem magnetic resonance imaging. Forensic science, medicine, and pathology. 2013;9(4):501-5. doi: 10.1007/s12024-013-9459-x.

13 Cha JG, Kim DH, Kim DH, Paik SH, Park JS, Park SJ, et al. Utility of postmortem autopsy via whole-body imaging: initial observations comparing MDCT and 3.0 T MRI findings with autopsy findings. Korean journal of radiology. 2010;11(4):395-406. doi: 10.3348/kjr. 2010.11.4.395.

14 Ruder TD, Thali MJ, Hatch GM. Essentials of forensic post-mortem MR imaging in adults. The British journal of radiology. 2014; 87(1036):20130567. doi: 10.1259/bjr.20130567.

15 Offiah CE, Dean J. Post-mortem CT and MRI: appropriate post-mortem imaging appearances and changes related to cardiopulmonary resuscitation. The British journal of radiology. 2016; 89(1058):20150851. doi: 10.1259/bjr.20150851.

Chapter 02

Fundamental aspects of X-ray computed tomography

2.1. Overview of CT physics

Conventional X-ray radiography projects three-dimensional (3D) body structures into a two-dimensional (2D) image, which leads to the loss of information regarding depth or thickness parallel to the X-ray (Fig. 1A).[1, 2]

Although 2D radiographs enable good visualization of high-contrast materials such as bone and air, they do not provide sufficient contrast to differentiate soft tissue structures because of superimposition caused by similar densities (e.g., when distinguishing the aorta from the heart or abdominal organs). To resolve these conventional radiography problems, X-ray CT has been introduced. It has gained popularity in various medical imaging fields (Fig. 1B). CT is an imaging procedure that typically uses a computer system and a rotating X-ray tube and detector assembly to produce cross-sectional images of the body (tomography) (Fig. 2).[3] By definition, tomography refers to any imaging technique that produces a sectional image of a selected plane in the body. Compared with conventional radiography, CT can provide depth information by producing 2D images from 2D thin-section data and stack those 2D images to create a gapless 3D image.[1] Current CT systems typically feature an X-ray tube and multiple detectors in an assembly that is mounted in a doughnut-shaped CT gantry; this rotates around the enclosed patient for data acquisition to create a sectional image.[2, 3] Subsequently, the patient is moved along the axis of the CT gantry to obtain another set of projection data from the next plane. The X-ray beam generated from the tube passes through a thin axial slice of the body, which continues at many different angles during the rotation of tube-detector assembly. On the opposite side of the tube, the detectors measure the X-ray that has passed through the body. Radiation transmission then enables the computer to calculate the degree of radiation absorption by using a large number of simultaneous equations of X-ray projection data, which are one-dimensional and acquired from many

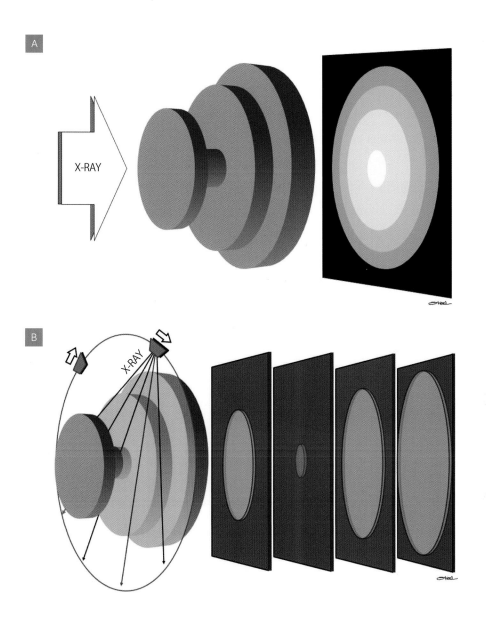

Figure 1. X-ray radiography and X-ray computed tomography (CT)
(A) Conventional X-ray radiograph projects three-dimensional structures into two-dimensional images, thereby losing depth information. (B) In contrast to conventional radiography, CT preserves depth information by producing a thin cross-sectional image of a selected plane through the target structure, eliminating tissue and organ overlap.

different directions in the chosen plane to produce the values of attenuation coefficients in each small voxel within a cross section.[1, 2] This information regarding the voxels is translated into a relative measure of radiodensity, known as the CT number or Hounsfield unit (HU).[2]

In the conventional CT method, the patient table does not move during scanning. It moves for subsequent scans during intervals between scans that are required for the stop/reverse rotation of the X-ray tube-detector assembly and respooling of the cables. A spiral CT (i.e., helical CT) system uses slip-rings (an electromechanical device), rather than electrical cables, to supply power; this allows the tube and detector to continue rotating while the patient moves perpendicular to the rotation plane. To increase the speed of image acquisition and volume coverage, multi-detector CT has been introduced as a form of

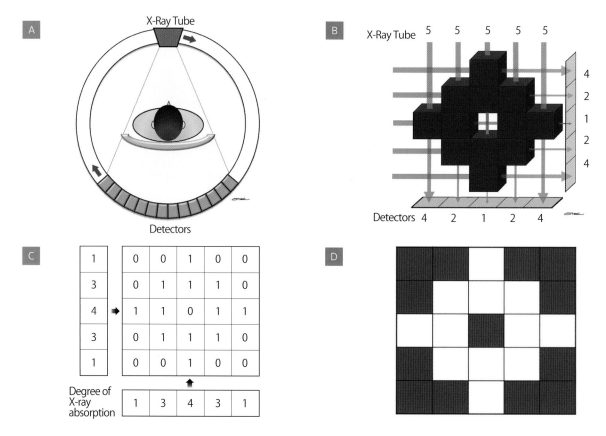

Figure 2. CT technique: How images are generated.
A CT system typically consists of an X-ray tube and detectors, which rotate around the enclosed patient for data acquisition to create a cross-sectional image (A). Detectors measure X-rays that have passed through the blocks (B), allowing the CT system to calculate the amount of X-ray attenuation in a sequential manner (C). Note the numbers in vertical and horizontal panels, which represent relative X-ray absorption by the blocks. Reconstruction of CT images is performed mathematically from a large number of X-ray projection data acquired at many different angles of the chosen plane, using traditional filtered back projection or more advanced iterative reconstruction techniques. This information regarding the voxels is translated into a relative measure of radiodensity, known as the CT number or Hounsfield unit (HU) (D).

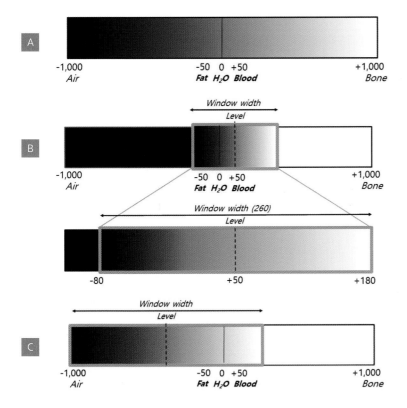

Figure 3. Transforming CT numbers to gray scale values.

(A) CT images consist of a wide range of CT numbers. In the Hounsfield scale, CT numbers are established with air as -1000 and water as 0. (B, C) The window level and width can be adjusted to examine a specific tissue of interest such as soft tissue (approximate WL of 50 HU and WW of 260 HU in b) or lung (approximate WL of -600 HU and WW of 1500 HU in C).

WW: window width, WL: window level.

spiral CT, which involves the conversion of a single row of detectors in the z-axis to multiple rows of detectors.[4]

2.2. Window width and Window level

CT images consist of a wide range of tissue densities, where air and water are defined as -1000 HU and 0 HU, respectively (**Fig. 3**). To view CT scans, windowing is required to transform HU numbers to gray scale values in a small subset of the overall dataset. This is used to improve the visualization of the particular structure of interest by increasing the contrast difference among tissues (**Fig. 4**). Windowing is con-

trolled by window width (WW) and window level (WL).[5] The WW is the measure of the range of CT numbers that are displayed in an image. The midpoint of the range is the WL, also referred to as the window center.[1, 5] The WW and WL can be changed to adjust the contrast and brightness of the image. For instance, a WL of 50 HU and a WW of 400 HU for better visualization of soft tissue will have a density range of −150 HU to +250 HU. In this scenario, any tissue with a density of −150 HU or less will be presented as black, and any tissue with a density of +250 HU or more will be presented as white on the CT image.

In general, standard axial CT views are viewed as if observing the body from below (**Fig. 5**), unless otherwise mentioned.

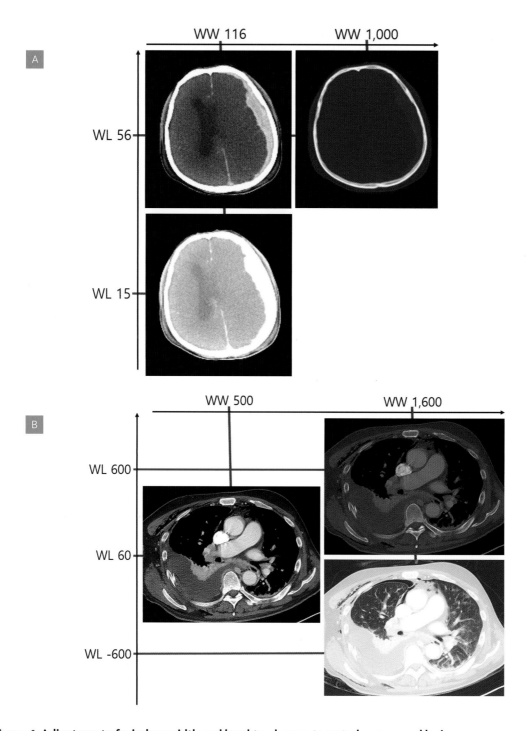

Figure 4. Adjustment of window width and level to observe targeted organs and lesions.
If the density value of an area is lower than the window level, that area becomes darker; when the density value exceeds the lower limit of the window width range, that area appears black. Wide window width exhibits an extensive range of tissue densities such as bones and lungs in an image, but involves the loss of discrimination of subtle density differences. Therefore, it becomes more difficult to differentiate between tissues with a narrow range of density values such as (A) white matter and gray matter in the brain and (B) soft tissue, blood, muscle, and fat.
WW: window width, WL: window level

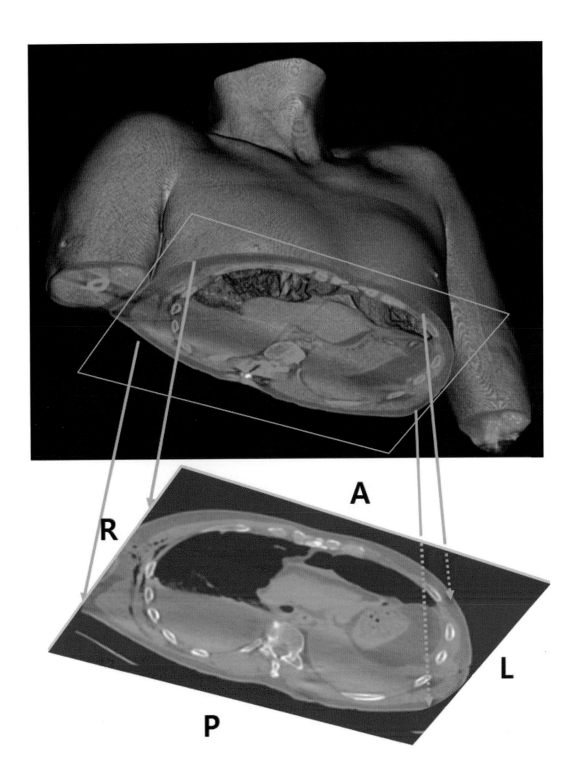

Figure 5. Standard axial CT view.
Examination of unprocessed source data displayed in the axial plane is necessary in clinical settings to obtain general overviews of lesions in terms of their presence, location, and type. Standard axial CT views are produced as if observing the patients from below, unless otherwise stated. A: anterior, P: posterior, L: left, R: right.

2.3. Postprocessing techniques

Image postprocessing refers to the use of various imaging techniques to generate additional images from axial raw data to highlight the necessary information and hide information that is not relevant to particular clinical findings.[6] Those techniques include multiplanar reconstruction (MPR) and various projection techniques that use "thickening" of MPR images. These include maximum intensity projection (MIP), minimum intensity projection (MinIP), and 3D volume-rendered (VR) approaches (**Figs. 6 and 7**).[7]

MPR refers to the process of using the original data stack obtained in a specific image plane, primarily axial, to create a 2D image in another plane. MPR images are generated from the original plane in either the coronal, sagittal, oblique, or curved plane--any plane with only one voxel thickness.[7, 8] Average intensity projection (AIP), also known as thick MPR, is created by averaging individual pixel densities--averaging the attenuation of each component in a selected section.[7] MIP images are created by showing voxels with the highest attenuation in the selected section. MIP is best used to improve the detection

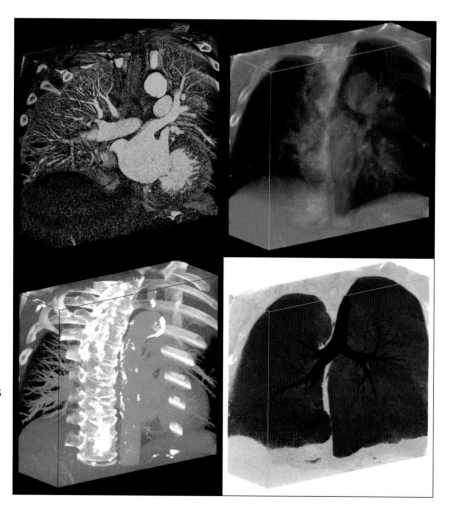

Figure 6. Multiplanar volume reformation images generated from the same original CT data. Clockwise from upper left, 3D VR, AIP (also known as thick multiplanar reconstruction), MinIP, and MIP images. All images were reconstructed with a slab thickness of 76 mm. VR: volume-rendered, AIP: average intensity projection (thick multiplanar reconstruction), MinIP: minimum intensity projection, and MIP: maximum intensity projection.

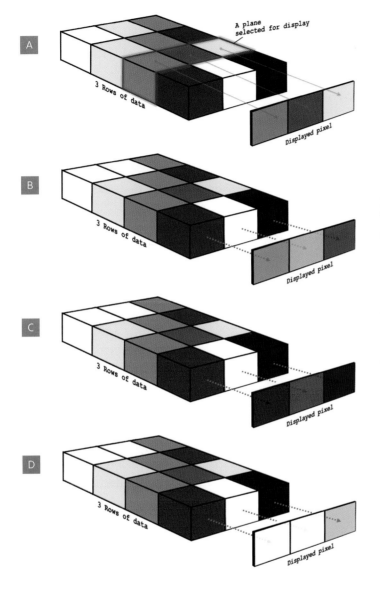

Figure 7. Multiplanar reformation and multiplanar volume reformation techniques.
The data consist of attenuation information expressed in Hounsfield unit values. The final projected value of the displayed two-dimensional pixel is determined by the processing algorithms and the amount of data selected for the calculation (i.e., slab thickness). MPR (A) refers to the process for generating nonaxial two-dimensional images from the axial CT data. These MPR images are produced from a plane with only one voxel thickness traversing a set of axial images in coronal, sagittal, oblique, or curved directions. Multiplanar volume reformations (B–D) use projection techniques for the thickening of multiplanar images. While AIP uses the mean Hounsfield unit values of the data to calculate the projected value in a slab (B), MinIP (C) and MIP (D) use only the lowest and highest voxel values found in the slab, respectively.
MPR: Multiplanar reformation, AIP: average intensity projection (also known as thick MPR), MinIP: minimum intensity projection, and MIP: maximum intensity projection.

of objects with the greatest attenuation in the image, such as contrast-filled vascular structures.[9, 10] MinIP operates in a similar manner to MIP, but images are produced by showing voxels with the lowest attenuation in the selected section. Therefore, MinIP can be used to show airways, areas of emphysema, or areas of abnormal air collection.[11] 3D VR is a group of techniques used to display a 2D projection of a 3D dataset, typically consisting of a stack of 2D slice im-

ages acquired by CT or MR imaging. VR provides a diagnostic benefit by combining 3D perspective with real-time interactive processing of the overall volume of sampled data for reconstruction.[7, 12]

The above techniques are easy-to-use tools for displaying the structures and lesions from various angles and perspectives after initial assessment using the standard axial plane.

References

1   Michael G. X-ray computed tomography. Phys Educ. 2001;36(6): 4426451. doi: 10.1088/0031-9120/36/6/301.

2   Goldman LW. Principles of CT and CT technology. Journal of nuclear medicine technology. 2007;35(3):115-28; quiz 29-30. doi: 10.2967/jnmt.107.042978.

3   Mahesh M. Search for isotropic resolution in CT from conventional through multiple-row detector. Radiographics: a review publication of the Radiological Society of North America, Inc. 2002;22(4):949-62. doi: 10.1148/radiographics.22.4.g02jl14949.

4   Goldman LW. Principles of CT: multislice CT. Journal of nuclear medicine technology. 2008;36(2):57-68; quiz 75-6. doi: 10.2967/jnmt.107.044826.

5   Xue Z, Antani S, Long LR, Demner-Fushman D, Thoma GR. Window classification of brain CT images in biomedical articles. AMIA Annual Symposium proceedings AMIA Symposium. 2012;2012: 1023-9.

6   B. FTO. Image Visualization and Post-processing Techniques. In: Multi-slice and Dual-source CT in Cardiac Imaging. Springer, Berlin, Heidelberg; 2007.

7   Dalrymple NC, Prasad SR, Freckleton MW, Chintapalli KN. Informatics in radiology (infoRAD): introduction to the language of three-dimensional imaging with multidetector CT. Radiographics: a review publication of the Radiological Society of North America, Inc. 2005;25(5):1409-28. doi: 10.1148/rg.255055044.

8   Rubin GD, Napel S, Leung AN. Volumetric analysis of volumetric data: achieving a paradigm shift. Radiology. 1996;200(2):312-7. doi: 10.1148/radiology.200.2.8685316.

9   Napel S, Marks MP, Rubin GD, Dake MD, McDonnell CH, Song SM, et al. CT angiography with spiral CT and maximum intensity projection. Radiology. 1992;185(2):607-10. doi: 10.1148/radiology. 185.2. 1410382.

10 Heath DG, Soyer PA, Kuszyk BS, Bliss DF, Calhoun PS, Bluemke DA, et al. Three-dimensional spiral CT during arterial portography: comparison of three rendering techniques. Radiographics: a review publication of the Radiological Society of North America, Inc. 1995;15(4):1001-11. doi: 10.1148/radiographics.15.4.7569120.

11 Ravenel JG, McAdams HP. Multiplanar and three-dimensional imaging of the thorax. Radiologic clinics of North America. 2003; 41(3): 475-89. doi: 10.1016/s0033-8389(03)00032-0.

12 Calhoun PS, Kuszyk BS, Heath DG, Carley JC, Fishman EK. Three-dimensional volume rendering of spiral CT data: theory and method. Radiographics: a review publication of the Radiological Society of North America, Inc. 1999;19(3):745-64. doi: 10.1148/radiographics. 19.3.g99ma14745.

Chapter 03

Postmortem CT and CT angiography - Technical consideration

3.1. Postmortem CT (PMCT)

Currently, PMCT is either performed using a dedicated CT scanner for postmortem use or a clinical CT scanner in the radiology department of the hospital.[1] Unrestricted radiation exposure, in combination with the absence of any motion-induced artifacts due to heartbeat and respiration, allows the acquisition of high-resolution image data that are required for the visualization of small structures or subtle injuries.[2, 3]

With the advances of CT technology in recent decades, most multi-detector CT scanners can produce thin slice images (approximately 1 mm thick) sufficient for imaging diagnosis. Therefore, without the implementation of dose reduction or motion correction algorithms, outdated CT scanners can be used in the postmortem setting.[4] However, in cases with subtle fractures of bones or rupture/occlusion of small vessels, slices of submillimeter thickness may be needed to localize those

pathologies.[1, 4] In addition, whole-body data acquisition is recommended, and a wide gantry opening is required when imaging larger corpses or those in an unusual body posture (**Fig. 1**). Therefore, a state-of-the-art CT scanner with advanced CT technology remains desirable in the postmortem setting.[1]

As in the clinical setting, PMCT images are generated from axial raw data using various postprocessing techniques in a workstation, such as multiplanar reconstruction (MPR), maximum intensity projection (MIP), or 3D volume-rendering (VR) techniques.[4, 5] Several commercially available workstations currently provide advanced postprocessing techniques and have been successfully translated into postmortem applications for image display and analysis.[4-6] For the review of the most cases, unprocessed axial source images yield a general overview regarding the presence, locations, and types of pathologies in areas of concern. Subsequently, MPR and MIP techniques are implemented as easy-to-use tools for enhanced visualization of the identified lesions from

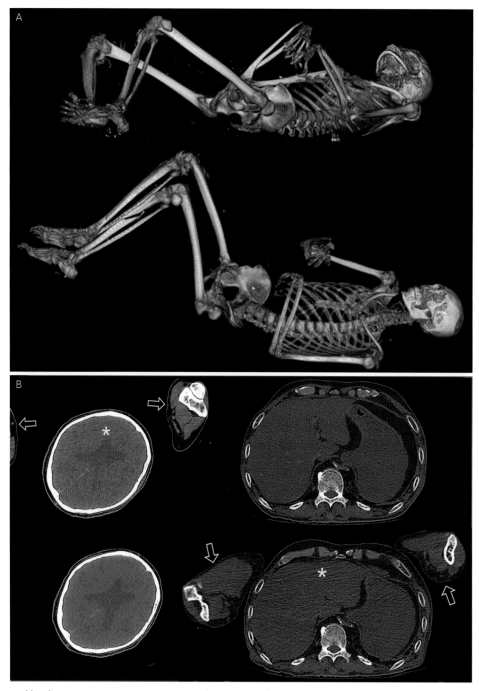

Figure 1. Effect of body posture on CT scanning and image quality.
(A) Three-dimensional volume-rendered images of a burned body show flexion of both legs and arms due to thermal retraction of muscles (i.e., heat-related change). This unusual body posture, along with obesity, often requires a wide gantry opening within the CT scanner. (B) Axial images of the CT scan of a body with the arms lifted up (top row) and down (bottom row) show streak artifacts (*) in the brain (top row) and abdominal cavity (bottom row), respectively. For postmortem CT scans, whole-body data acquisition is typically performed; therefore, both upper arms are inevitably included in the scan field. Their presence in the scanning field leads to streak artifacts in some views, which may degrade image quality.

various angles and perspectives beyond primary assessment of the standard axial plane. Manually created curved MPR images can also be used to follow the course of vascular structures, particularly coronary arteries. Accordingly, MPR, MIP, and other comparable techniques (e.g., 3D VR and curved MPR) show lesions more intuitively, and provide concise diagnostic information in a few corresponding images.[7] Three-dimensional VR images may be more tolerable to the public or in court, and may provide a more intuitive understanding of the mechanism of injuries in traumatic casualties (**Fig. 2**).[1]

However, a major hurdle for the widespread application of PMCT as a regular pre-autopsy procedure is its failure to provide detailed vascular information, particularly in natural cardiovascular deaths, the most common cause of unexpected deaths at coronial autopsy. To address this concern, PMCT with intravascular contrast medium injection (PMCT angiography; PMCTA) has been adopted, and it has shown encouraging results for the direct visualization of vascular abnormalities such as occlusion and rupture.[4, 5, 8]

3.2. Postmortem CT angiography (PMCTA)

The first angiography of an amputated hand was performed using a radiopaque mixture consisting of lime, cinnabar (mercury), and petroleum in 1896. Subsequently, various contrast materials were explored for postmortem angiography using conventional radiography in the first half of the 20th century.[9, 10] These materials include corpuscular

preparations (e.g., barium sulfates, bismuth chloride, lead sulfate, or potassium iodine), casts (e.g., silicon rubber or microfilm), and water-soluble Gastrografin® for separate ex vivo or in vivo evaluations of a single organ, such as the heart.[5, 11] Since the implementation of CT in forensic death investigations, considerable effort has been directed to the development of contrast agents suitable for the postmortem vascular environment: absence of circulation without heartbeat, increased permeability of vascular walls, and collapsed vascular lumen (empty or partially filled with postmortem clots and gas).[11, 12] Therefore, the vessels must be flushed and expanded with an adequate volume of contrast material for sufficient visualization of the entire vascular system. However, the greatest challenge has been to identify suitable contrast materials to cope with the increased vascular permeability that develops after death.

In the era of PMCT, most materials developed in the early 20th century are no longer used. Currently, hydrophilic (water-soluble) and lipophilic (lipid-soluble) iodinated solutions are the most frequently used contrast materials for the combination of PMCT and postmortem angiography used to generate PMCTA. Numerous techniques for the injection of contrast into the vascular system have been developed to examine individual organs (e.g., coronary arteries of the ascending aorta, either isolated or in situ) or to visualize the entire vasculature through whole-body CT angiography. This whole-body visualization is becoming increasingly popular. Regardless of their water-solubility or lipid-solubility, contrast agents can change the chemical compositions of body fluid samples. Therefore, samples of interest should be col-

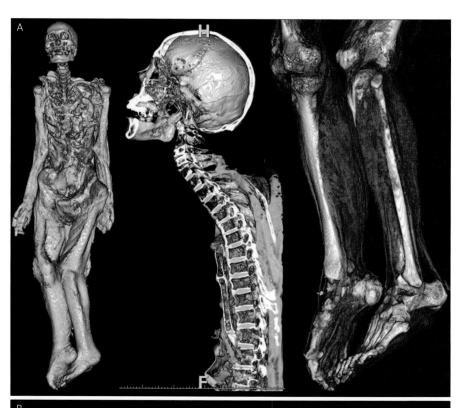

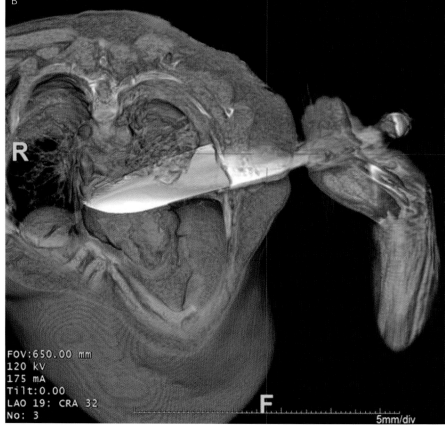

Figure 2. Three-dimensional (3D) volume-rendered (VR) display of postmortem CT images.

(A) Postmortem CT of a 73-year-old male found dead. 3D VR images provide a quick, at-a-glance view of the overall state of the body and show unbalanced decomposition of the head and trunk. Note the presence of almost intact muscles and tendons under the skin of both legs. (B) A female victim of domestic violence. In this fatal stabbing case, 3D CT images provide insights regarding the penetration distance and direction of a knife without autopsy photographs.

lected for biochemical studies before contrast injection when toxicological examinations of body fluids (e.g., blood and urine) are required to determine the cause of death.

3.2.1. Water-soluble contrast agent

Although widely used in the clinical setting, water-soluble iodinated agents cannot be directly applied to whole-body PMCTA due to the extensive increase in vascular permeability after death. The use of intravascular hydrophilic agents causes rapid fluid extravasation through hyperpermeable vascular walls that leads to histological artifacts of surrounding tissue and incomplete expansion of vascular lumens. To overcome this limitation, Jackowski et al. proposed the addition of hygroscopic polyethylene glycol (PEG) as a contrast agent dissolver and volume expander, which could reduce the speed of extravasation by increasing the viscosity of the hydrophilic contrast mixture.[13] Currently, the most popular composition of hydrophilic mixture for PMCTA is an iodized contrast medium (hydrophilic monomer) mixed with PEG 200 (larger polymer) at a ratio of 1:10. [4] After injection of the contrast mixture, enhancement is found prominently in hypervascular solid organs (e.g., cerebral and cerebellar cortices, heart, liver, and kidneys), as in clinical imaging (**Fig. 3**).[8]

This parenchymal enhancement originates from the extravascular diffusion of smaller hydrophilic iodized molecules, while large hygroscopic PEG molecules remain in the vessel. In contrast to lipid-soluble contrast agents, the extravascular diffusion of iodinated components after injection of this mixture leads to a gradual decrease in the level of vascular enhancement and thus allows separate observations of arterial and venous systems at short (20-min) intervals between arterial and venous injections. Accordingly, the delay between injection and scanning should be no ≤20 min when a water-soluble mixture is used.[4, 8] Furthermore, a previous report and our own experience indicate that the hydroscopic properties of the contrast mixture tend to induce the clumping of blood remaining in the vessels; this involves pulling water from surrounding tissue and could obscure a thrombosis.[1, 11]

3.2.2. Lipid-soluble contrast agent

In contrast to water-soluble agents, oily liquids mostly remain in the vascular lumen and occlude capillary beds (e.g., during hepatoma chemoembolization using lipiodol. {ethyl ester of iodized poppy seed oil, Guerbet AG} in the clinical setting).[11, 14] When used for postmortem angiography, the vessel diameter that can be filled by oily liquids depends on the liquid viscosity. Therefore, when the liquid viscosity is excessive, optimal contrast enhancement cannot be achieved in organ parenchyma due to the extensive blocking of contrast into microcapillary beds. In contrast, when the liquid viscosity is insufficient, extensive leakage of contrast into organs is observed, especially at sites of early autolysis (e.g., pancreas or gastric mucosa) (**Fig. 4**).[3, 5, 8, 15]

These agents flush out postmortem clots and do not mix with remaining blood, thus yielding high-contrast images and enabling estimation of the extravasated amount of blood during autopsy.[3, 11] Another advantage of oily liquids is that they can remain within the vasculature for at least 72 h (**Fig. 5**).[8, 16]

This is useful in a case with scan delay after injection or in bodies with advanced decomposition (Fig. 6).

However, oily liquid may infiltrate the damaged vessel walls and dislodge lipids from atherosclerotic plaques, altering the size and shape of plaque morphology.[5] Furthermore, oily liquid can mimic pulmonary fat embolisms. Therefore, tissue sampling may be necessary to determine the cause of death in cases where fat embolism is suspected (e.g., multiple traumas).[17, 18] Standard formulas of these contrast agents comprising mixtures of oily perfusates and iodized oil are actively in use for PMCTA. Initially, lipiodol was used for oily contrast and low-viscosity diesel oil was used for both perfusion and volume expansion. Recently, esters of poly-iodinated fatty acids (i.e., Angiofil®, Fumedica AG, Muri, Switzerland) have been introduced for dedicated forensic use, and the combination of Angiofil and medium-viscosity paraffin oil (paraffinum liquidum) has become a popular alternative to oil-based contrast solutions for

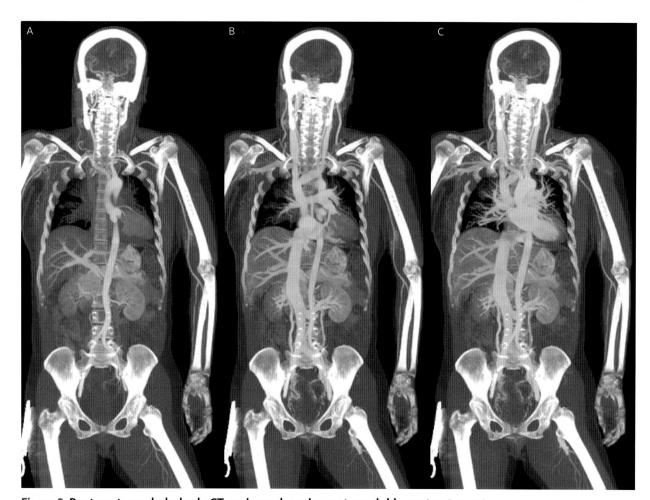

Figure 3. Postmortem whole-body CT angiography using water-soluble contrast agent.
Coronal maximum intensity projection images with a slab thickness of 70 mm. Arterial (A), venous (B), and dynamic (C) phases.

performing PMCTA worldwide.[18]

3.2.3. Contrast-injection technique

A unilateral femoral approach is used to inject contrast media into the vascular system. After skin incision, one cannula is inserted into the femoral artery and another cannula is inserted into the femoral vein, allowing separate retrograde injection of contrast into the arterial system and antegrade injection into the venous system.[4, 5, 8] Without the

aid of a heartbeat, contrast medium must be forcefully injected into partially collapsed blood vessels using a mechanical pump. Various types of pumps are currently used. For example, centrifugal pumps (e.g., an embalming machine), roller pumps for precise control of pressure and injection volume, and/or custom-designed injectors to support individual needs on an institutional basis **(Fig. 7)**.[1, 4, 11, 19]

In this chapter, we introduced whole-body PMCTA techniques using water-soluble and lipid-

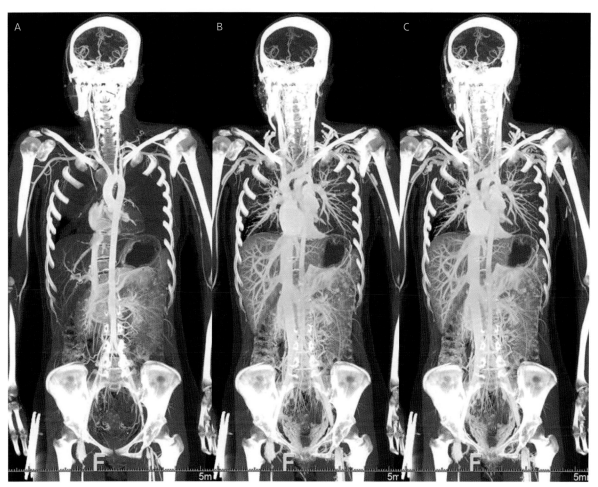

Figure 4. Postmortem whole-body CT angiography using lipid-soluble contrast medium.
Coronal maximum intensity projection images with a slab thickness of 58 mm. Arterial (A), venous (B), and dynamic (C) phases.

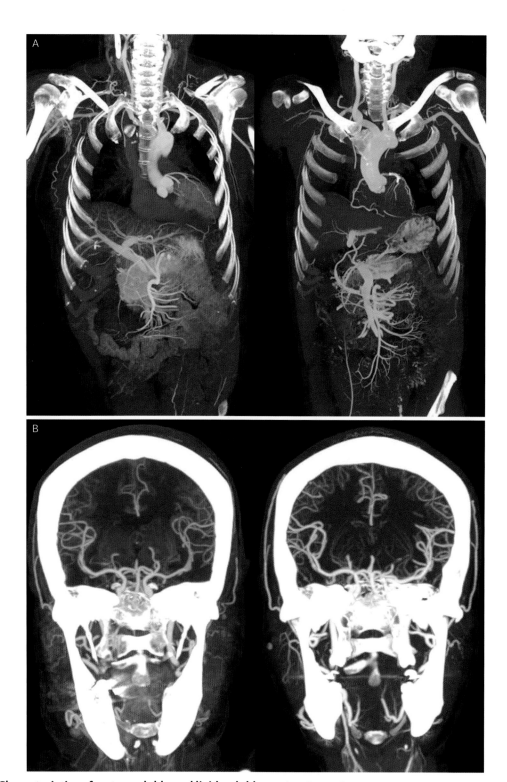

Figure 5. Characteristics of water-soluble and lipid-soluble contrast agents.
Maximum intensity projection images in the arterial phase of postmortem CT angiography of trunk (A) and head (B) using water-soluble (left in A and B) and lipid-soluble contrast agent (right in A and B), respectively. Note the prominent enhancement of brain parenchyma and myocardium by rapid contrast extravasation when water-soluble agent was used.

soluble contrast agents. Many studies have shown that PMCTA enables adequate visualization of the vascular system with the injection of a water-soluble mixture of PEG and hydrophilic contrast agent (i.e., an agent currently used in the clinical setting) using a basic flow-calibrated roller or centrifugal pump. [4, 20] The protocol consists of successive scanning of arterial and venous systems after separate injections of 1,500 mL and 1,800 mL at 600 mL/min to localize the bleeding source. Usually, the first injection is administered into the arterial system, followed by the venous system; the opposite cannula remains open to ensure pressure equalization within the capillary bed. When water-soluble contrast media are used to investigate coronary artery disease, the body should be in the prone position to assure adequate filling of the ascending aorta and right coronary artery, because these contrast agents are heavier than any

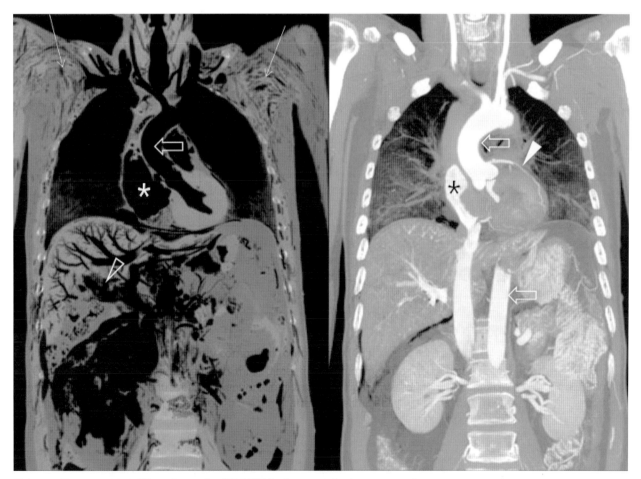

Figure 6. Postmortem CT angiography (PMCTA) of a severely decomposed case.
Minimal intensity projection image (left) of postmortem CT shows extensive putrefactive gases (long arrows) throughout the body, including the cardiac chamber (*), aorta (arrow), and portal veins (arrowheads). Postmortem CT angiography was successfully performed in this case and a reconstructed maximum intensity projection image (right) demonstrates the contrast-filled cardiac chambers and vascular structures, including aorta (arrows) and coronary artery (white arrowhead).

residual blood.[4]

To inject a lipid-soluble contrast agent, multiphase PMCTA has been introduced, consisting of four phases. Specifically, nonenhanced PMCT is followed by three injections of a mixture of 6% lipid-soluble Angiofil® and paraffin oil: an arterial (1,200 mL at 800 mL/min) phase injection, venous (1,800 mL at 800 mL/min) phase injection, and finally, additional arterial injection of 500 mL to the arterial system at 200 mL/min; the venous system is maintained open to allow spontaneous drainage (dynamic phase injection). The initial two injections are used to fill

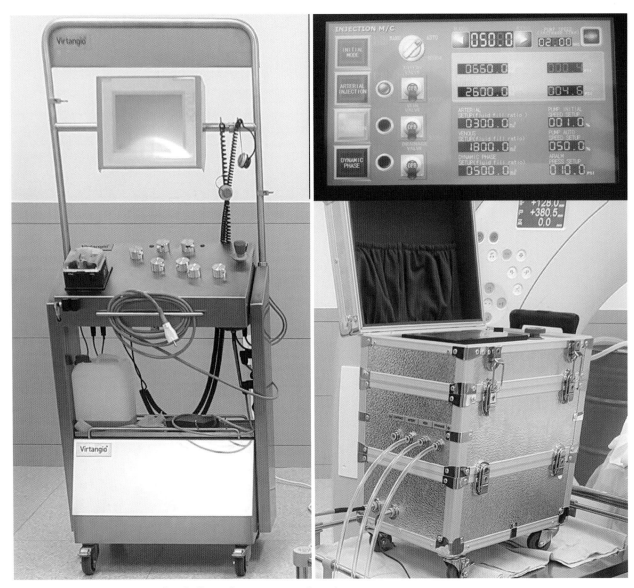

Figure 7. Contrast injectors for dedicated postmortem imaging.
Injection pumps used for postmortem CT angiography. Virtangio machine (left) and AngelBox–portable centrifugal pump (right).

the arterial and venous systems, whereas subsequent dynamic phase injection is performed to confirm the diagnosis by comparing its findings with findings from the other two phases. Similar to injection methods for water-soluble agents, two cannulas are placed into the femoral artery and vein after a skin incision is made in the unilateral inguinal area.[18] These two cannulas are then connected to an injection pump (e.g., a basic centrifugal pump or dedicated roller pump) for meticulous volume or pressure control to inject the lipid-soluble contrast medium needed for each angiographic phase (Fig. 8).

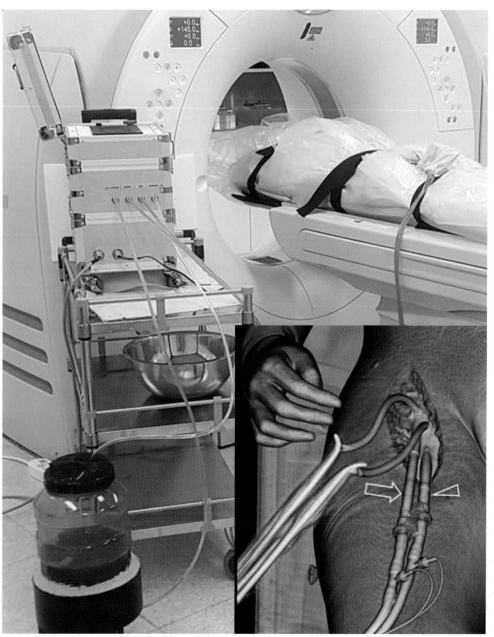

Figure 8. Postmortem CT angiography using a custom-designed centrifugal injection pump.
Contrast mixture is injected separately into the femoral artery and femoral vein through two individual arterial (arrow) and venous lines (arrowhead).

References

1. Lee H, Lee S, Cha JG, Baek T, Yang KM. Postmortem Computed Tomography and Computed Tomography Angiography: Cardiothoracic Imaging Applications in Forensic Medicine. Journal of thoracic imaging. 2019;34(5):286-98. doi: 10.1097/rti.0000000000000398.

2. Lundström C, Persson A, Ross S, Ljung P, Lindholm S, Gyllensvärd F, et al. State-of-the-art of visualization in post-mortem imaging. APMIS: acta pathologica, microbiologica, et immunologica Scandinavica. 2012;120(4):316-26. doi: 10.1111/j.1600-0463.2011.02857.x.

3. Grabherr S, Egger C, Vilarino R, Campana L, Jotterand M, Dedouit F. Modern post-mortem imaging: an update on recent developments. Forensic sciences research. 2017;2(2):52-64. doi: 10.1080/20961790. 2017.1330738.

4. Ross SG, Bolliger SA, Ampanozi G, Oesterhelweg L, Thali MJ, Flach PM. Postmortem CT angiography: capabilities and limitations in traumatic and natural causes of death. Radiographics: a review publication of the Radiological Society of North America, Inc. 2014; 34(3):830-46. doi: 10.1148/rg.343115169.

5. Grabherr S, Grimm J, Dominguez A, Vanhaebost J, Mangin P. Advances in post-mortem CT-angiography. The British journal of radiology. 2014;87(1036):20130488. doi: 10.1259/bjr.20130488.

6. Lee H, Park H, Cha JG, Lee S, Yang K. Myocardial Contrast Defect Associated with Thrombotic Coronary Occlusion: Pre-Autopsy Diagnosis of a Cardiac Death with Post-Mortem CT Angiography. Korean journal of radiology. 2015;16(5):1024-8. doi: 10.3348/kjr.2015. 16.5.1024.

7. Schoepf UJ, Zwerner PL, Savino G, Herzog C, Kerl JM, Costello P. Coronary CT angiography. Radiology. 2007;244(1):48-63. doi: 10.1148/radiol.2441052145.

8. Ross S, Spendlove D, Bolliger S, Christe A, Oesterhelweg L, Grabherr S, et al. Postmortem whole-body CT angiography: evaluation of two contrast media solutions. AJR American journal of roentgenology. 2008;190(5):1380-9. doi: 10.2214/ajr.07.3082.

9. Haschek E, Lindenthal T. Ein Beitrag zur Praktischen Verwerthung der Photographie nach Röntgen. Wien Klin Wochenschr. 1896;9: 63-4.

10. Busch U. Wilhelm Conrad Röntgen: The Discovery of X-rays and the Creation of a New Medical Profession. In: Russo P, editor. Handbook of X-ray Imaging: Physics and Technology. Boca Raton: CRC Press; 2017. p. 327-30.

11. Grabherr S, Grimm J, Baumann P, Mangin P. Application of contrast media in post-mortem imaging (CT and MRI). La Radiologia medica. 2015;120(9):824-34. doi: 10.1007/s11547-015-0532-2.

12. Michaud K, Grabherr S, Doenz F, Mangin P. Evaluation of postmortem MDCT and MDCT-angiography for the investigation of sudden cardiac death related to atherosclerotic coronary artery disease. The international journal of cardiovascular imaging. 2012;28(7): 1807-22. doi: 10.1007/s10554-012-0012-x.

13. Jackowski C, Bolliger S, Aghayev E, Christe A, Kilchoer T, Aebi B, et al. Reduction of postmortem angiography-induced tissue edema by using polyethylene glycol as a contrast agent dissolver. Journal of forensic sciences. 2006;51(5):1134-7. doi: 10.1111/j.1556-4029.2006. 00207.x.

14. Nakakuma K, Tashiro S, Hiraoka T, Uemura K, Konno T, Miyauchi Y, et al. Studies on anticancer treatment with an oily anticancer drug injected into the ligated feeding hepatic artery for liver cancer. Cancer. 1983;52(12):2193-200. doi: 10.1002/1097-0142(19831215) 52: 12<2193::aid-cncr2820521203>3.0.co;2-r.

15. Bruguier C, Mosimann PJ, Vaucher P, Uské A, Doenz F, Jackowski C, et al. Multi-phase postmortem CT angiography: recognizing technique-related artefacts and pitfalls. International journal of legal medicine. 2013;127(3):639-52. doi: 10.1007/s00414-013-0840-9.

16. Grabherr S, Djonov V, Yen K, Thali MJ, Dirnhofer R. Postmortem angiography: review of former and current methods. AJR American journal of roentgenology. 2007;188(3):832-8. doi: 10.2214/ajr. 06. 0787.

17. Schneider B, Chevallier C, Dominguez A, Bruguier C, Elandoy C, Mangin P, et al. The forensic radiographer: a new member in the medicolegal team. The American journal of forensic medicine and pathology. 2012;33(1):30-6. doi: 10.1097/PAF.0b013e31820c6aa3.

18. Grabherr S, Doenz F, Steger B, Dirnhofer R, Dominguez A, Sollberger B, et al. Multi-phase post-mortem CT angiography: development of a standardized protocol. International journal of legal medicine. 2011;125(6):791-802. doi: 10.1007/s00414-010-0526-5.

19. Schweitzer W, Flach P, Thali MJ, Laberke P, Gascho D. Very economical immersion pump feasibility for postmortem CT angiography. J Forensic Radiol Imaging. 2016;5:8614. doi: 10.1016/j.jofri. 2015.11.009.

20. Ross SG, Thali MJ, Bolliger S, Germerott T, Ruder TD, Flach PM. Sudden death after chest pain: feasibility of virtual autopsy with postmortem CT angiography and biopsy. Radiology. 2012;264(1): 250-9. doi: 10.1148/radiol.12092415.

Traumatic Death

The entire universe need not arm itself to crush him:
A vapour, a drop of water suffices to kill him.
– Blaise Pascal, 1623–1662.

Chapter 04

Blunt force trauma

4.1. Introduction

Blunt force trauma, also known as non-penetrating injury, is defined as physical trauma to the body resulting from forceful impact with a blunt object or flat surface.[1] It is one of the most common types of trauma leading to serious injury and is frequently observed by forensic pathologists in the investigation of traumatic death.[2] Fatal blunt force injury commonly involves almost all types of transport accidents (e.g., motor vehicle collision, pedestrian hit by a vehicle or railway train, and aviation crashes) (Fig. 1), jumps or falls from height, and blows from a blunt object without any sharp edge (e.g., a fist, baseball bat, or ball).[1, 2] (Fig. 2).

Head injury is the most common cause of traumatic death in motor vehicle accidents, followed by extremities and thoracic injuries.[1-4] However, other types of injuries such as burn, blast, sharp force injury, drowning, and asphyxiation may be superimposed on, or combined with, underlying blunt force injury. In those instances, the cause of death is difficult to determine. Furthermore, people who have died of natural causes often exhibit comparatively minor blunt force injuries (i.e., to skin or soft tissue) that would not have contributed to death (Fig. 3). In some instances, fatal blunt trauma can be combined with mild pre-existing natural disease that would not directly cause death but may lead to fatal traumatic injuries.

Therefore, when investigating trauma-related death, care must be undertaken to identify underlying or newly developed natural diseases. Consideration should then be given to the relative severities and causal relationships of those potential causes of death (e.g., cerebral aneurysmal rupture that leads the victim to fall from height).

The current gold standard for forensic examination in trauma-related deaths is autopsy dissection, which allows for inspection, palpation, and the direct visualization of major injuries that may contribute to death. However, the main limitations of autopsy are its subjective and observer-dependent nature. In addition, standard autopsy procedures involve extensive mutilation of the body that can potentially change topographic relationships and destroy delicate findings, thus causing problems in second opinion or re-examination.[5-8] Because of its ability to demonstrate bony fractures, foreign bodies, and abnormal gas collection, Postmortem CT (PMCT) is a useful noninvasive adjunct in cases of blunt trauma, including traffic accidents, falls from heights, or violent assaults. Multiplanar and three-dimensional (3D) reconstruction of the head, trunk, spine, and extremities enhance our intuitive understanding of the mechanism and type of injuries, providing figurative depictions of the pattern and relationship of injuries before autopsy dissection (**Figs. 3 and 4**).[9] Furthermore, in cases with internal bleeding, the density of blood changes over time before death. CT aids in estimating the age of blood at the time of death, based on its change in density during the evolution of hemorrhage.[10] (see Chapter 11 for details)

PMCT angiography (PMCTA) is reportedly useful for pre-autopsy assessment of vascular injuries that are inaccessible or can be exposed solely through extensive tissue mutilation during autopsy. PMCTA allows the demonstration of vascular narrowing, obstruction, or rupture in cases of natural cardiovascular deaths. In cases of traumatic death, PMCTA is also suitable for evaluating vascular injuries and localizing the source of hemorrhage from blunt injuries (e.g., traffic accidents, falls from heights, and violent assaults), which is difficult and time-consuming or impossible by conventional autopsy.[6-9]

4.2. Head Injuries

Blunt head trauma occurs from non-penetrating impact of a blunt object or from a sudden movement of the head.[11] The common causes are motor vehicle accidents and falls, followed by sports injuries and physical assaults.[12] The damage from direct impacts comprises scalp laceration, soft tissue injury, bony fractures, intracranial hemorrhage (ICH), or brain parenchymal contusions. Acceleration or deceleration injury by abrupt shaking of the head has been presumed to result in subdural hemorrhage or diffuse axonal injuries, although this remains a source of controversy.

A skull fracture occurs when an impact to the head is sufficiently forceful to break the cranial bones. Although linear fracture is the simplest type of fracture and occurs with low impacts or blows to the head (**Fig. 5**), skull fractures may become more complex depending on the angle, location, and force of an impact; these complex fractures include circular, stellate, comminuted (broken into three or more sections), and depressed types (**Fig. 6**).[1]

Trauma is the leading cause of intracranial hemorrhage (ICH) and may lead to direct or indirect damage to arteries and veins beneath the skull. This damage causes intracranial, extraparenchymal, or intraparenchymal hemorrhage.[13] ICH includes four types of hemorrhage: epidural hemorrhage (EDH), subdural hemorrhage (SDH), subarachnoid hemorrhage (SAH), and hemorrhagic contusion of the brain.[14] Hemorrhagic contusions are most frequently caused by substantial head impact and motion, with or without combined skull fracture. They

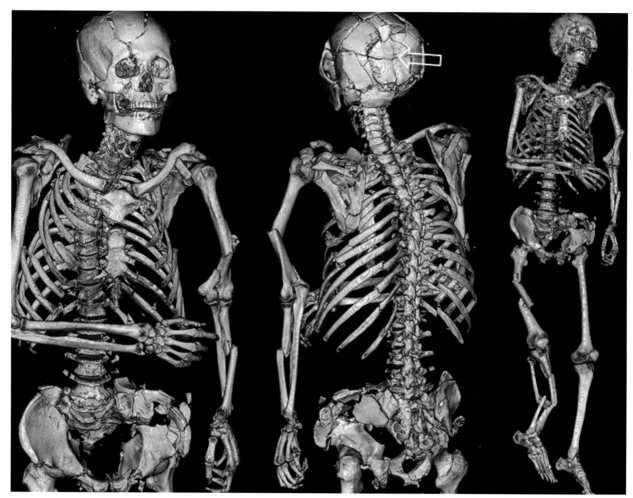

Figure 1. A pictorial representation of complex traumatic injury in a victim of fall from height and run-over accident.
Three-dimensional figurative images of postmortem CT with a volume-rendered technique enhance intuitive understanding of the injury pattern and mechanism by demonstrating the relationships among bony fragments in fatal trauma. Note the spiderweb fracture of vertex and high occiput (arrow), a pattern characteristic of fall-related fatal injury.

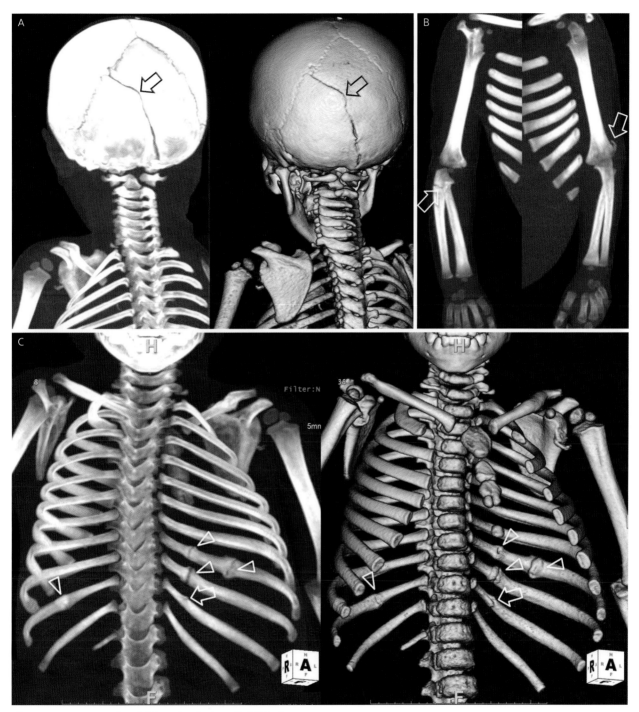

Figure 2. A 16-month-old female victim of child abuse.
Three-dimensional volume-rendered (right in A and C) and maximum intensity projection images of postmortem CT demonstrate multifocal bony fractures in the skull (arrow in A), humerus, ulna (arrows in B), and ribs (arrow in C). Note multiple rib fractures in multiple stages of healing (arrowheads in C).

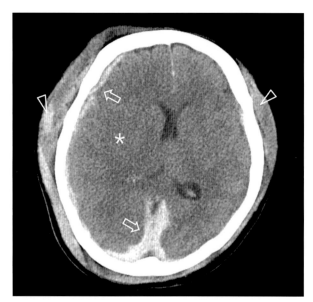

Figure 3. A 39-year-old female who died of acute cerebral infarction.
Antemortem CT shows cortical hypodensity with associated parenchymal swelling and a loss of corticomedullar junction in right middle cerebral artery territory, suggesting acute cerebral infarction (*). Note the presence of SDH in the right frontal area (arrow) and bilateral occipital areas with scalp swelling (arrowheads) and hematoma on the right fronto-temporo-occipital and left temporal areas, presumably due to secondary trauma related to cerebral infarction.

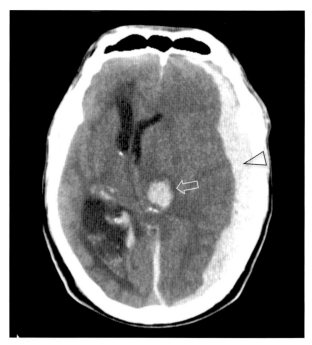

Figure 4. Hypertensive intracranial hemorrhage and secondary traumatic SDH.
Antemortem CT demonstrated focal hypertensive intracranial hemorrhage (arrow) on the left thalamus, which might have led to subsequent traumatic subdural hematoma (arrowhead) in the ipsilateral left hemisphere.

begin as small foci of petechial hemorrhage that may be combined into larger parenchymal hematomas. These contusions are predominantly located on the crest of a gyrus in the anterior and posterior temporal lobes, as well as the inferior frontal lobes, adjacent to the overlying bony protuberance.[15] Hemorrhagic contusions are caused by focal microvascular injuries in which the brain parenchyma collides with the overlying skull. These injuries frequently occur under the site of impact (coup injury) or on the side of the brain directly opposite to the area of impact (contrecoup injury), particularly in severe cases (**Figs. 7**

and 8).[1, 13]

SDH is a collection of blood at the junction of the dura and arachnoid, which commonly occurs after tearing of the bridging veins that course in the subdural space. Although commonly regarded as subdural, this is a potential space in the dural border cell layer, which is dissected open by extravasated blood or cerebrospinal fluid and does not naturally.[16] SDHs are most commonly caused by blunt head trauma and acceleration-deceleration injuries (**Figs. 8 and 9**).

SDHs are often associated with cerebral cortical

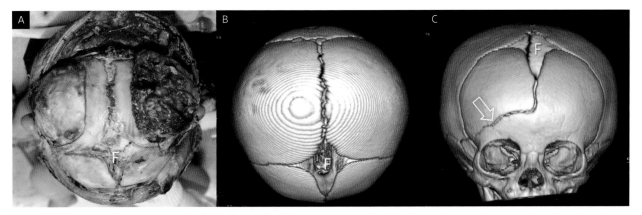

Figure 5. A transverse fracture not found during autopsy.
Autopsy photograph of the skull observed from above (A). A three-dimensional volume-rendered (3D VR) image corresponding to the left image (B). A 3D VR image viewed from the front (C). A linear skull fracture immediately above the right superior orbital rim was not identified during autopsy (arrow), due to the limited range of scalp dissection from the calvarium. F: anterior fontanelle.

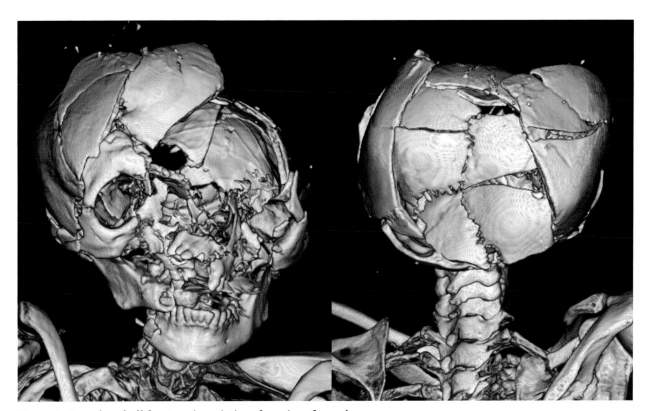

Figure 6. Complex skull fracture in a victim of an aircraft crash.
Three-dimensional volume-rendered images show a complex pattern of comminuted bony fractures in great detail, including depressed fractures of the vertex and spiderweb fractures of the occiput. This image was taken without removing the body from the body bag.

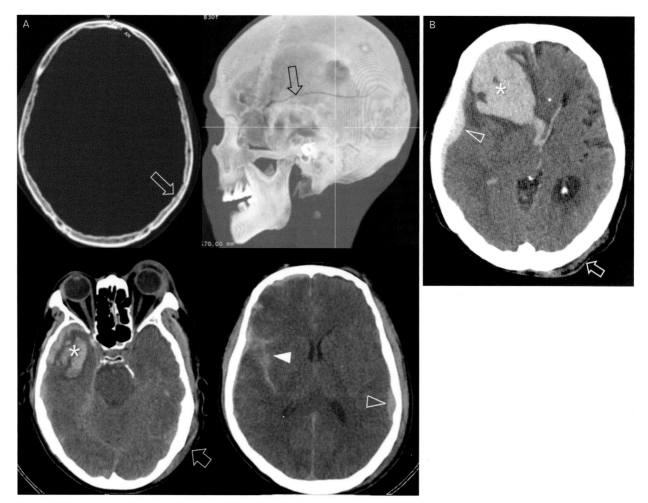

Figure 7. Two cases of traumatic contusion of the brain cortex, combined with subdural hematoma (SDH).
(A) A 53-year-old male with a fatal slip-and-fall injury after drinking. Postmortem CT depicts a linear skull fracture (arrows) with focal scalp hematoma (short arrow) and SDH (arrowhead) on the left temporoparietal area. Note the presence of subcortical contusion (*) in the right temporal lobe and subarachnoid hemorrhage (white arrowhead) in the Sylvian fissure as a contrecoup injury. (B) CT of fatal slip-and-fall injury in a 73-year-old female. She had a primary forceful impact on the left posterior parietal area. Note the presence of focal scalp hematoma on the left posterior parietal and occipital areas (arrow) of the head as a primary impact. Consequent contrecoup injuries on the right frontal area consist of a massive subcortical parenchymal contusion (*) on the right frontal lobe and localized subdural hemorrhage (arrowhead).

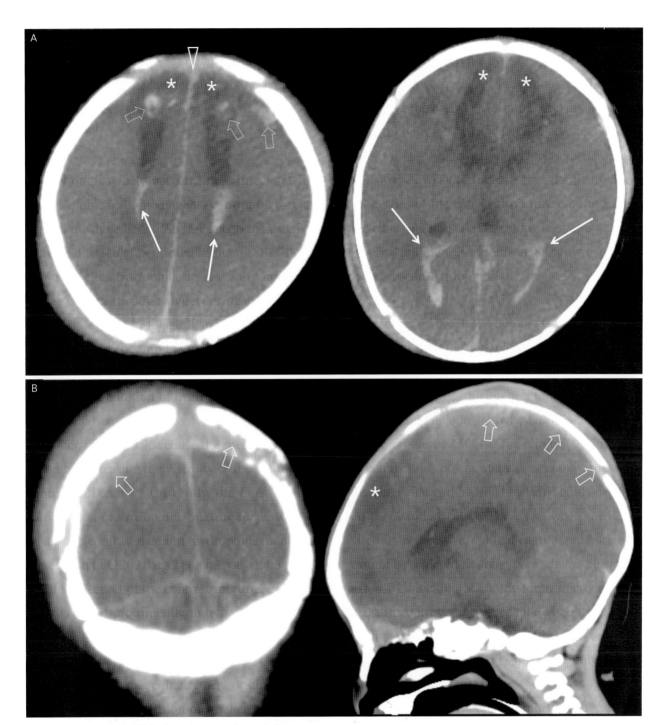

Figure 8. A case of child abuse in a newborn infant.
(A) Axial CT shows acute hemorrhagic contusions (arrows) with surrounding leukomalacia (*) in the subcortical areas of both frontal lobes; it also depicts interhemispheric hemorrhage (arrowhead) and intraventricular hemorrhage (long arrows). These findings raise suspicion of multistage injuries of the brain. (B) Coronal (left) and parasagittal (right) images demonstrate acute subdural hemorrhage (arrows) of bilateral parietal areas and leukomalacia (*) of the subcortical area of the frontal lobe.

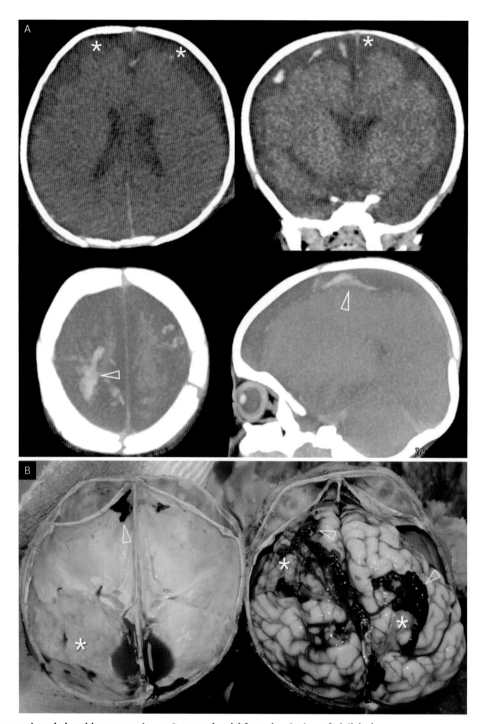

Figure 9. Traumatic subdural hygroma in an 8-month-old female victim of child abuse.
(A) Axial (upper left) and coronal (upper right) images of PMCTA show fluid collection in the subdural space of the frontal area. The subdural fluid has a low density similar to ventricular fluid (*); axial (lower left) and sagittal (lower right) images with maximum intensity projection also show multifocal high densities inside (arrowheads) the collected subdural fluid. These findings suggest a subdural hygroma that could have caused a rapid increase in intracranial pressure due to recent bleeding. (B) Specimen photographs show thin membranes previously containing the hygroma in the subdural space (*). Note the presence of multiple blood clots (arrowheads) corresponding to high-density areas on the CT image.

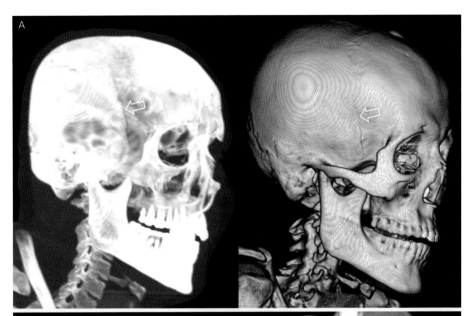

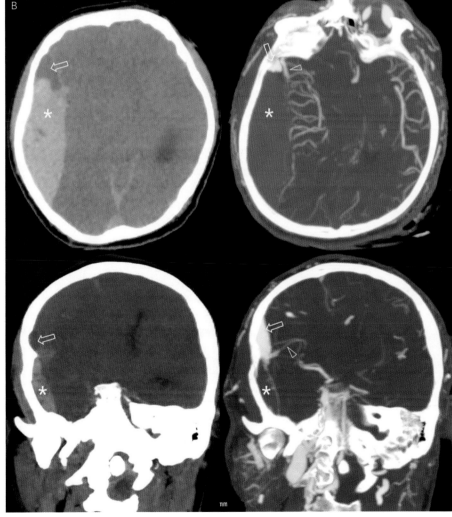

Figure 10. Traumatic epidural hemorrhage (EDH) caused by the rupture of an anterior branch of the middle meningeal artery in a 35-year-old male.
(A) MIP (left) and three-dimensional volume-rendered images (right) show a linear skull fracture in the right temporal area, which is frequently associated with EDH. (B) Axial (left upper) reformation and coronal (left lower) MIP images of postmortem CT show lentiform-shaped hemorrhage with internal high density (*) in the right temporoparietal area, which corresponds to the acute stage of an EDH. EDH generally tends to appear lenticular with a comparatively short length and thick width, due to the requirement for peeling the dural attachment from the suture. Note the presence of focal low-density areas (arrows in left upper and left lower) in the hematoma, which provide evidence of hyperacute nonclotted blood. After intra-arterial contrast injection, axial (right upper) and coronal (right lower) MIP images identify the site of rupture by depicting active leakage of contrast agent from the anterior branch of the middle meningeal artery, which then accumulates in the low-density area (arrows in left upper and left lower) of acute EDH. Note that cortical vessels are medially displaced by the hematoma (right upper).
MIP: Maximum Intensity Projection

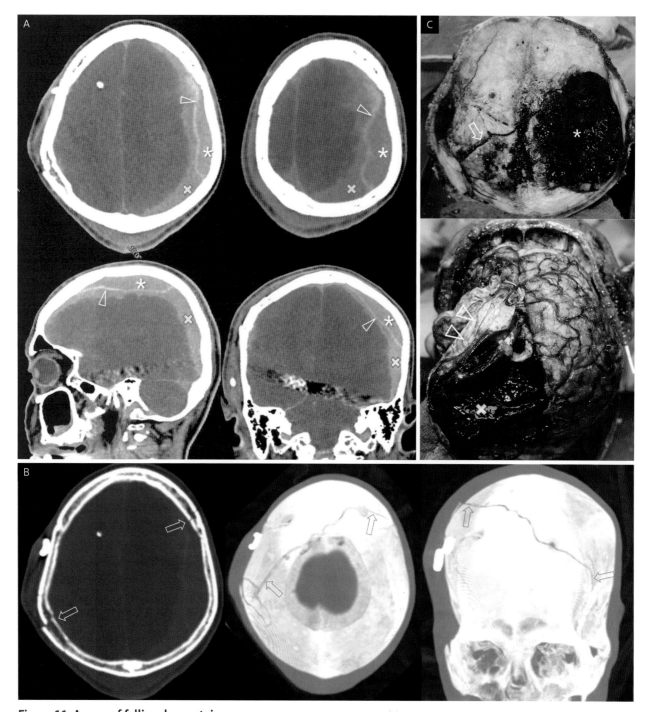

Figure 11. A case of falling down stairs

(A) Axial (upper row), sagittal (lower left), and coronal (lower right) images of postmortem CT show both EDH (*) and SDH (x) located on the outside and inside of the dura mater (arrowhead) in the left temporoparietal area, respectively. (B) Linear skull fracture (arrow) is noted from the right parietal area to the left frontotemporal area of the calvarium. (C) Autopsy photograph of the calvarium demonstrates EDH (*) on the surface of the inner calvarium (upper) and SDH (X) beneath the dura (arrowhead) in the lower image. Note the presence of a linear fracture (arrow) of the right parietal bone. Currently, EDH is presumed to result from direct trauma, whereas SDH is presumed to result from damage to cortical bridging veins due to brain recoil. See Ind J Neurotr. 2008;5:113-114 and Asian J Neurosurg. 2012;7(4):210-213.
EDH: epidural hematoma, SDH: subdural hematoma

injuries; in many cases, clinical features depend on the site and severity of those injuries.[14] The dura mater consists of periosteal, meningeal, and dural border cell layers. EDH is a collection of blood in the epidural space between the skull and periosteal dura.[16] Bleeding is caused mostly by traumatic laceration of an artery (e.g., the middle meningeal artery in the subdural space) and often accompanied by associated skull fracture **(Fig. 10)**.

These EDH lesions tend to be lenticular in shape and do not cross the suture lines because they are constrained by tight dural attachment at the sutures.[16] Although less common than SDH, this is a life-threatening condition because high-pressure bleeding secondary to arterial injury may result in more rapid hematoma growth and deadly increases in intracranial pressure.[14] EDHs are usually coup injuries that occur under a site of direct impact either by blood leakage from a skull fracture or injury to the menin geal arteries. In contrast, SDHs are frequently contrecoup lesions that arise from venous injuries. Although it is not very common, some patients with severe head trauma develop EDH and SDH on the same side **(Fig. 11)**.

SAH is defined as the extravasation of blood into the subarachnoid space between the arachnoid membrane and the pia mater, both of which cover the brain. This hemorrhage is the result of injury to the vessels coursing through the subarachnoid space. Overall, SAH is most commonly caused by traumatic injury to the brain, but it can be caused spontaneously by the rupture of a cerebral aneurysm or by an arteriovenous malformation.[13, 17] When an individual dies unexpectedly after sustaining comparatively minor blunt trauma to the head (e.g., a single punch), a potential explanation for that death involves traumatic injury to the vertebral artery. Although some deaths after minor blunt trauma might result from a fall to the ground, thus leading to skull fractures or intracranial hemorrhage, most of these deaths are caused by basal SAH. Subsequent vertebral artery injury is regarded as the major vascular pathology in those assault-related deaths **(Figs. 12-14)**. However, the direct visualization of a vertebral artery injury may not always be possible. On the basis of the difficult location and time-consuming destructive dissection of this area, pathological conditions (e.g., dissection, ruptures, intimal damage, or thrombus formation of vertebral arteries) that could be related to the death are difficult to diagnose and often not investigated during a standard autopsy dissection. PMCTA suggested traumatic vertebrobasilar injury in all cases in our study, demonstrating arterial perforation, luminal irregularity, and occlusion.

4.3. Injuries to the body trunk

Motor vehicle accidents comprise the majority of blunt injuries to the trunk, together with falls from heights and work-related accidents. Blunt trauma to the trunk involves a wide spectrum of injuries such as soft tissue contusion, bony fractures, and organ injuries (e.g., heart, major vessels, lungs, diaphragm, and abdominal organs).[1]

Traumatic injuries to the bony thorax frequently occur in combination with pneumothorax, hemothorax, and lung injuries. In these instances, rib

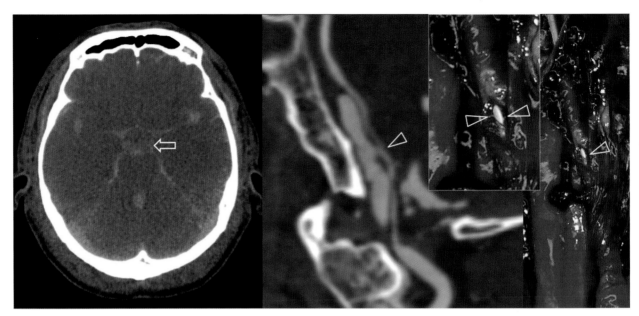

Figure 12. A 59-year-old male victim of domestic violence.
Axial image of PMCT depicts a typical basal subarachnoid hemorrhage (arrow in left panel) and curved MPR image of postmortem CT angiography (middle) demonstrates focal perforation of the left vertebral artery with contrast extravasation (arrowhead) to the subarachnoid space. Pathology specimen photos (right) confirm a focal rupture of V_4 Segment in the left vertebral artery (arrowheads). PMCT: postmortem CT, PMCTA: postmortem CT angiography, MPR: multiplanar reformation.

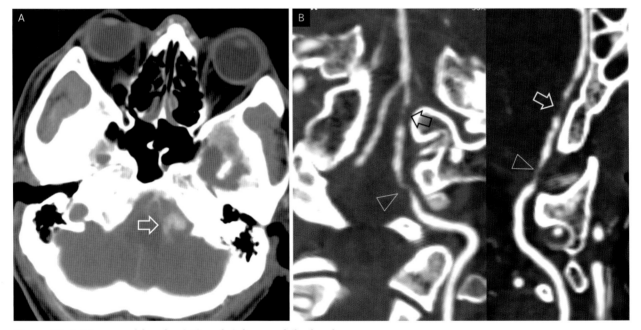

Figure 13. A 46-year-old male victim of violence while drunk.
Axial image of contrast-enhanced antemortem CT (A) performed at the emergency department shows basal subarachnoid hemorrhage and focal rupture of the left vertebral artery (arrow), which were confirmed on curved multiplanar reformation images of postmortem CT angiography (B) as luminal narrowing and irregularity (arrows). Another potential vascular injury (arrowheads) is evident on the distal segment of the left vertebral artery, but was not evident during clinical CT examination.

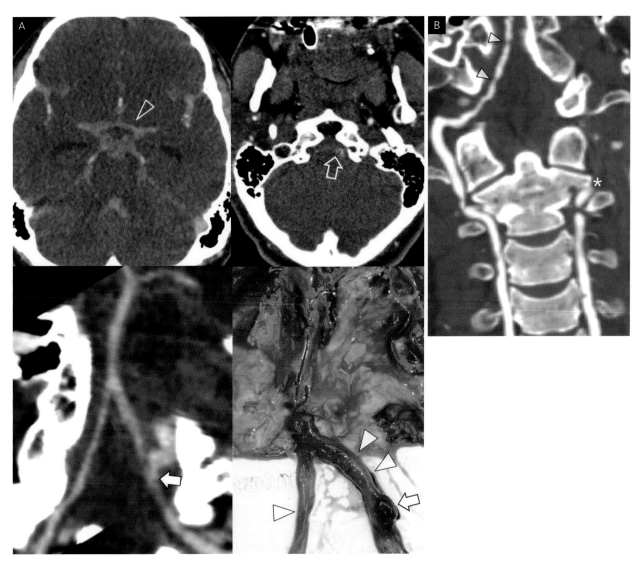

Figure 14. A 40-year-old male hit on the head while drunk.
(A) Antemortem clinical CT shows subarachnoid hemorrhage (arrowhead) at the basal cistern on a nonenhanced image
(left upper) and a focal rupture of the left vertebral artery (arrows) on axial (right upper) and curved MPR images (left
lower) of contrast-enhanced CT. Pathology specimen (right lower) confirms a focal rupture of the vertebral artery (arrow)
and diffuse and focal thrombi (arrowheads) in the right and left vertebral artery, respectively. (B) Curved MPR image
of postmortem CT angiography shows no contrast filling in the left vertebral artery, suggesting complete occlusion
of the left artery with thrombosis (*) and diffuse luminal irregularity of the distal segment of the right vertebral artery
(arrowhead). MPR: multiplanar reformation.

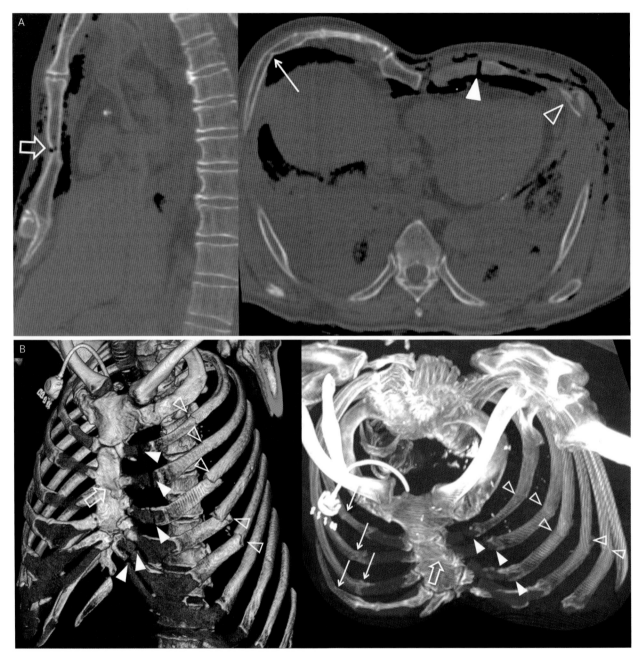

Figure 15. Multiple rib fractures and a sternal fracture related to vigorous cardiopulmonary resuscitation (CPR).
Sagittal (left) and axial (right) multiplanar reconstruction image (A). 3D VR image (left) and MIP image (right) (B).
(A) Postmortem CT images reveal symmetrical distribution of fractures of left rib (arrowhead) and costal cartilage (white arrowhead) and deformity (long arrow) of the right rib at anterior angle as well as sternal fracture (arrow), characteristic of CPR-related injuries. (B) Multiple deformities of the right ribs (long arrows) and transverse fractures of the sternum body (arrows) as well as fractures of left ribs (arrowheads) and costal cartilage (white arrowheads) are also depicted on 3D VR (left) and MIP (right) images, which aid in the intuitive understanding of the lesion distribution.
3D VR: Three-dimensional volume-rendered, MIP: Maximum Intensity Projection.

fractures are usually associated with chest wall hemorrhage and sternal fractures are typically found at the third intercostal space as a form of transverse fracture. In contrast, cardiopulmonary resuscitation-related fractures are usually found at the anterior angles of ribs and lower sternum (**Fig. 15.**).[1, 18, 19]

In motor vehicle accidents, blunt force injuries with direct compressive force to chest and upper abdomen are common when the steering wheel and dashboard hit the drivers. Furthermore, the sudden deceleration of the body may push the heart and aorta to the anterior chest and result in tearing of the aortic isthmus, where the aorta is tightly attached to the mediastinum by the ligamentum arteriosum (**Fig. 16**).[1]

Heart injury is less common than aortic injury in motor vehicle accidents. Depending on the severity of impact forces, it includes a spectrum of injury patterns: myocardial contusion, laceration, and rupture, as well as pericardial lacerations. Cardiac injuries may be accompanied by hemopericardium, hemomediastinum, or hemothorax. Hemopericardium may lead to cardiac tamponade and cause death with a fatal accumulation of at least 150 mL of blood in the pericardial cavity.[20]

Although injuries to abdominal organs usually do not cause death, they can be accompanied by multisystem trauma to the body, contributing to morbidity and mortality. However, in cases of strong impact force to the abdomen, massive peritoneal or retroperitoneal hemorrhage may cause death from laceration or rupture of the visceral organs (e.g., liver, spleen, pancreas, and kidneys) and major abdominal vessels. Splenic injuries occur frequently with rib fractures because of force to the left upper abdomen (**Fig. 17**).

Hepatic injuries may occasionally be associated with rib fractures. Renal contusion or rupture occur with blunt force to the flank.[1] Although rare, pancreatic injury occurs mostly in connection with polytrauma after motor vehicle accidents in adults, bicycle handlebar strikes in children, or violence in both groups.[21, 22] Injury to the pancreas is usually subtle and difficult to identify by imaging modalities. Therefore, it is associated with substantial morbidity and mortality in the event of overlooked diagnosis (**Fig. 18**).[22]

Pelvic hemorrhage is the most severe fatal complication of pelvic fractures, an important consequence of blunt injuries to the pelvis. Active bleeding remains the major cause of death in patients with pelvic fractures. Hemorrhage may originate from arteries and veins (e.g., branches of the iliac artery or major pelvic veins) that are damaged by or within the fractured bony fragments.[23]

4.4. Spine and other skeletal injuries

Blunt force injuries to the spine and other bony structures include skin and soft tissue injuries, bony fractures, and dislocations. Trauma with excessive impact (e.g., by motor vehicle, pedestrian, aviation, and diving accidents) often results in the most severe forms of injury and death (**Fig. 19-21**).

Fatal hemorrhage from vascular tearing or cord injuries, mostly vertebral fracture-related compression or transection, may cause immediate death

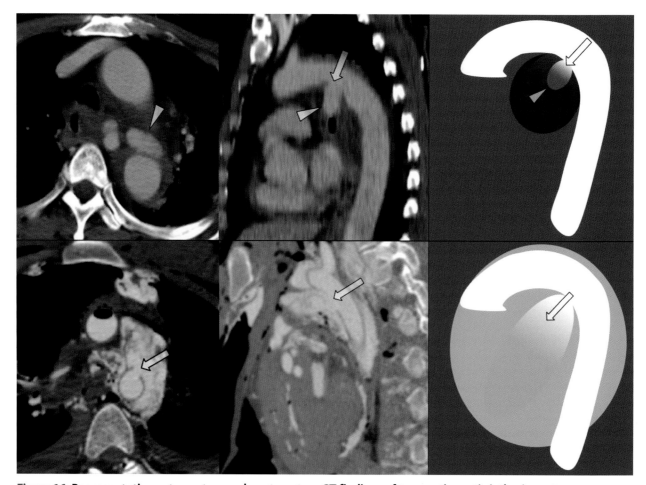

Figure 16. Representative antemortem and postmortem CT findings of traumatic aortic isthmic rupture.
Upper row: clinical CT angiography of a 57-year-old male pedestrian victim. Axial (left) and oblique sagittal (middle) images with corresponding schematic illustration (right). Lower low: PMCTA of a motorbike rider killed in a road accident. Axial (left) and oblique sagittal (middle) images with corresponding schematic illustration.
(upper row) As a sign of vital reaction, active adenosine triphosphate-consuming coagulation forms a barrier against contrast leakage through the defect (arrows), appearing as a saccular luminal outpouching (arrowheads) that manifests as a pseudoaneurysm. Lower row: conversely, after death, contrast leaks through the defect (arrows) in the aortic wall and spreads freely into the adjacent mediastinal space, due to the lack of vital reaction - coagulation process.

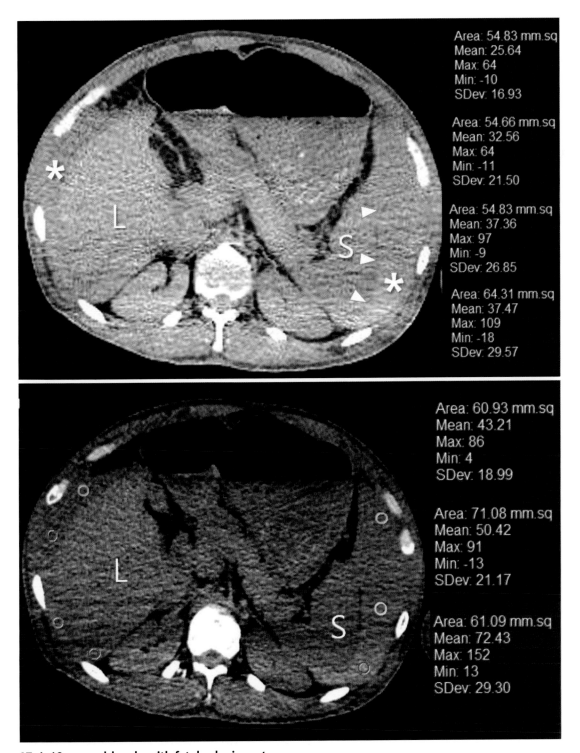

Figure 17. A 40-year-old male with fatal splenic rupture.
Postmortem axial CT images show that a higher hemorrhage density (*) has accumulated near the spleen (43-72 HU) than near the liver (26-37 HU), which raises the suspicion of splenic injury as a source of hemorrhage. Hemorrhage collects near the bleeding source at early stages of bleeding; it can be identified by the high-density fluid on nonenhanced CT (arrowheads), which is regarded as the "sentinel clot sign". Autopsy confirmed the splenic rupture.

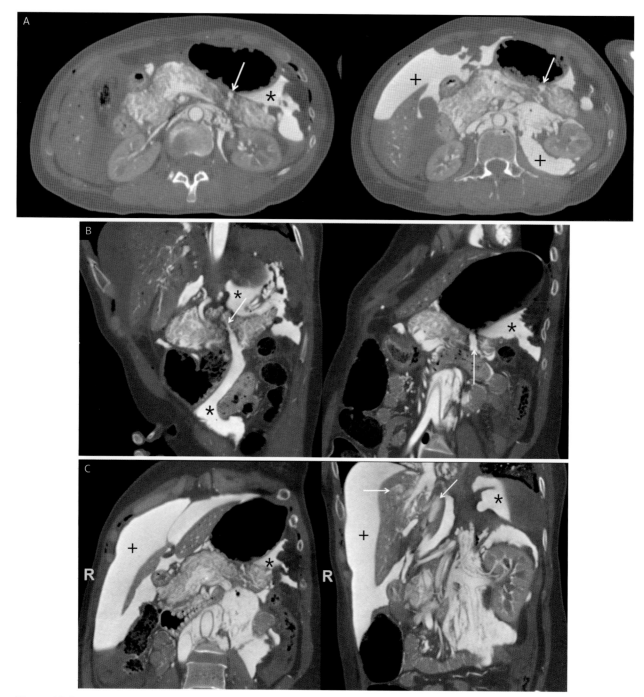

Figure 18. Postmortem CT angiography of a 48-year-old female victim of a violent assault.
(A) Axial images obtained after contrast injection into arterial (left) and then venous (right) systems show fracture of the pancreatic body (arrows) and arterial bleeding (*) into peripancreatic and perisplenic spaces, as well as venous bleeding (+) into perihepatic and perirenal spaces. (B) Oblique coronal (left) and oblique sagittal (right) images after arterial injection show direct contrast leakage (*) from the pancreatic fracture. (C) Oblique coronal images obtained after subsequent venous injection of contrast medium show massive venous bleeding (+) into perihepatic and perisplenic spaces, without evidence of gross large vein injuries. Note the presence of hepatic parenchymal hemorrhages, consistent with traumatic contusion of the liver.

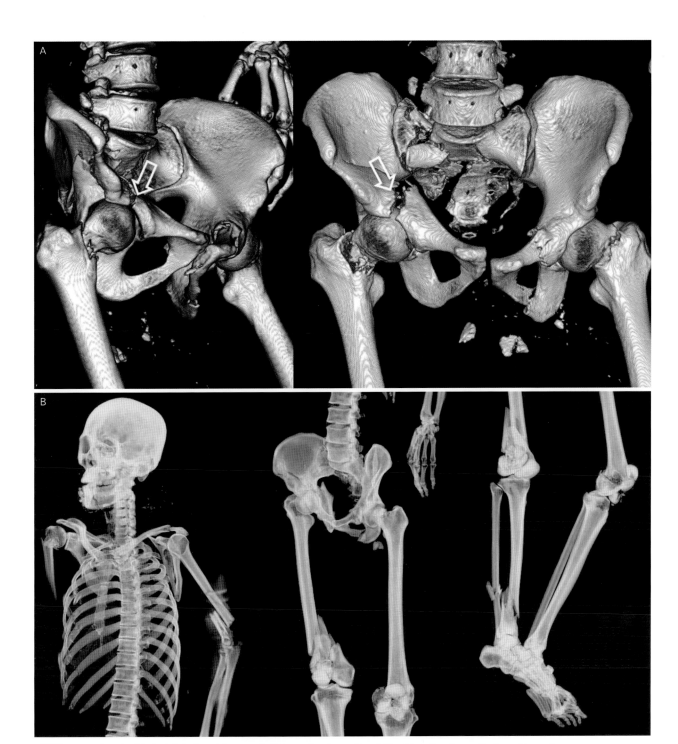

Figure 19. Acetabular fracture and femoral dislocation in a pilot killed in a fatal small aircraft crash.
Three-dimensional volume-rendered images of postmortem CT demonstrate multiple fractures of the pelvic bones, sacrum, femoral heads and necks, and right acetabulum (A) as well as ribs, left radius, and right distal femur, tibia, and fibula (B). Pelvic injuries have been found in victims of motor vehicle accidents. However, acetabular fractures are not frequently observed in the clinical setting; they mainly occur after high-energy impacts (e.g., falls from heights or high-speed car accidents), which are known to cause polytraumatic injuries with a high mortality rate.

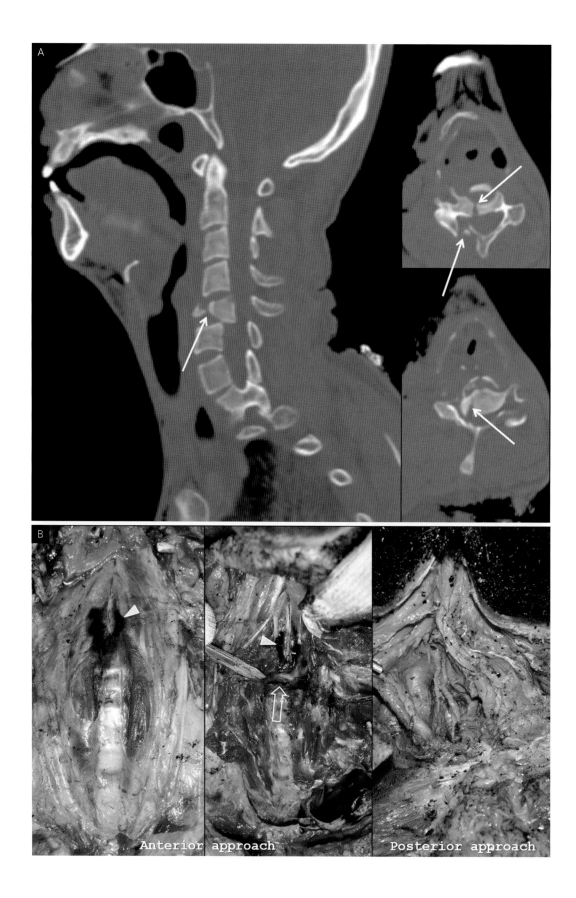

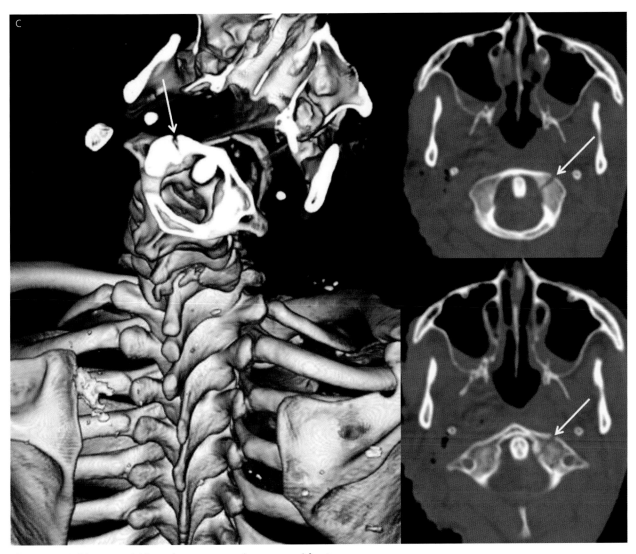

Figure 20. A 29-year-old female passenger in a car accident.
Sagittal (left) and axial (right) images (A) of postmortem CT show hyperflexion fractures (long arrows) of the C5 vertebral body, which (arrow) were easily detected with adjacent hemorrhage (arrowheads) through an anterior approach during autopsy dissection (left and middle images in b). However, no deeper dissection was made because no soft tissue hemorrhage was found upon superficial incision of the posterior neck (right image in B), preventing identification of the Atlas fracture. In contrast, three-dimensional volume-rendered image (left in C) and axial images (right in C) show fracture of the left anterior position of the lateral mass of the C1 vertebral body (long arrows); these structures are difficult to approach during routine autopsies. C5: 5th cervical

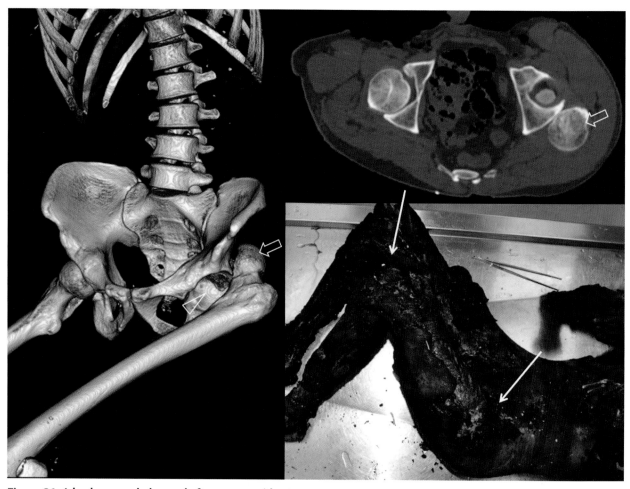

Figure 21. A body severely burned after a car accident.

Three-dimensional volume-rendered image (left) and axial image (upper right) show dislocation of the left femoral head (arrows) from the acetabular fossa (arrowhead). The body was severely burned after a traffic accident. Autopsy photograph shows heat-related changes in body posture, including flexion of lower limbs due to thermal retraction of the muscles. Because of this flexion deformation of the thigh, damage to the pelvis was not identified during the autopsy. However, femur head dislocation was easily identified with the use of CT imaging.

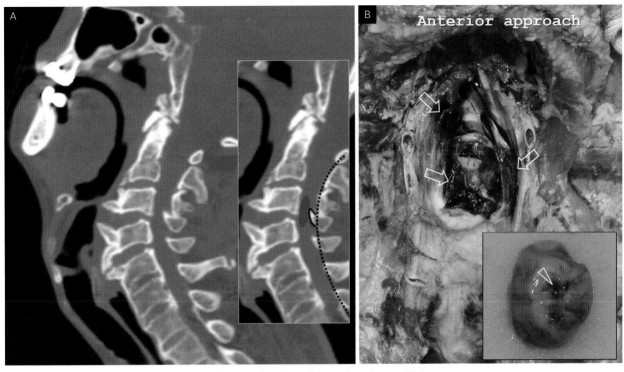

Figure 22. A passenger who died in a traffic accident involving a head-on collision.
(A) Sagittal image of postmortem CT shows retrolisthesis of the third cervical vertebral body on the fourth body; the potential mechanism of injury to the spinal cord (red ellipsoid) by the bony structure (edged in black) is depicted in the magnifying box. (B) Photograph of the autopsy specimen shows hemorrhage in the soft tissue (arrows) surrounding the cervical spine and spinal cord (arrowhead). While CT cannot detect a small amount of soft tissue and spinal cord hemorrhage, spinal alignment may change during autopsy dissection and is therefore difficult to assess. This case shows that PMCT is a useful noninvasive adjunct to autopsy in cases of blunt trauma, and that it can be performed without opening the body and modifying anatomical relationships.

after trauma. Pulmonary thromboembolism, fat embolism, and infection are frequent complications that may cause delayed death during treatment. Recent implementation of various CT reconstruction techniques can help to establish the types of bony fractures, force direction, and mechanism of injury, particularly in the event of spinal injury, using 3D pictorial representation.[9] Although PMCT detects bony fractures more accurately, a substantial proportion (20%) of lethal spinal cord injuries are reportedly found only during autopsy, without CT abnormalities (**Fig. 22**).

Therefore, accurate assessment of spinal trauma may require the use of both CT and autopsy. MR imaging can also be used to assess cord injury.[24]

References

1. Levy A, Harcke T. Blunt force injury. Essentials of Forensic Imaging: A Text-Atlas 1st ed. Boca Raton: CRC Press; 2010. p. 97-116.

2. Prahlow JA, Byard RW. Blunt Force Injury Deaths. In: Prahlow JA, Byard RW, editors. Atlas of Forensic Pathology. Humana Press; 2012. p. 389-486.

3. Kaewlai R, Avery LL, Asrani AV, Novelline RA. Multidetector CT of blunt thoracic trauma. Radiographics: a review publication of the Radiological Society of North America, Inc. 2008;28(6):1555-70. doi: 10.1148/rg.286085510.

4. Swierzewski MJ, Feliciano DV, Lillis RP, Illig KA, States JD. Deaths from motor vehicle crashes: patterns of injury in restrained and unrestrained victims. The Journal of trauma. 1994;37(3):404-7.

5. Saukko P, Knight B. The forensic autopsy. In: Saukko P, editor. The Knight's Forensicc Pathology. 3rd ed. London: CRC press; 2004. p. 1-47.

6. Ross SG, Bolliger SA, Ampanozi G, Oesterhelweg L, Thali MJ, Flach PM. Postmortem CT angiography: capabilities and limitations in traumatic and natural causes of death. Radiographics: a review publication of the Radiological Society of North America, Inc. 2014; 34(3):830-46. doi: 10.1148/rg.343115169.

7. Chevallier C, Doenz F, Vaucher P, Palmiere C, Dominguez A, Binaghi S, et al. Postmortem computed tomography angiography vs. conventional autopsy: advantages and inconveniences of each method. International journal of legal medicine. 2013;127(5):981-9. doi: 10.1007/s00414-012-0814-3.

8. Grabherr S, Grimm J, Dominguez A, Vanhaebost J, Mangin P. Advances in post-mortem CT-angiography. The British journal of radiology. 2014;87(1036):20130488. doi: 10.1259/bjr.20130488.

9. Lee H, Lee S, Cha JG, Baek T, Yang KM. Postmortem Computed Tomography and Computed Tomography Angiography: Cardiothoracic Imaging Applications in Forensic Medicine. Journal of thoracic imaging. 2019;34(5):286-98. doi: 10.1097/rti.0000000000000398.

10. Ruder TD, Zech W, harcke GM, Ross S, Ampanozi G, Thali MJ, et al. Still frame from the hour of death: Acute intracerebral hemorrhage on post-mortem computed tomography in a decomposed corpse. J Forensic Radiol Imag. 2013;1(2):73-6. doi: 10.1016/j.jofri.2013.03.042.

11. Martin RM, Wright MJ, Lutkenhoff ES, Ellingson BM, Van Horn JD, Tubi M, et al. Traumatic hemorrhagic brain injury: impact of location and resorption on cognitive outcome. Journal of neurosurgery. 2017;126(3):796-804. doi: 10.3171/2016.3.jns151781.

12. Haydel M, Burn sB. Blunt Head Trauma..[Updated 2020 Aug 10] StatPearls.[Internet] Treasure Island (FL): StatPearls Publishing; 2020 Jan-.

13. Heit JJ, Iv M, Wintermark M. Imaging of Intracranial Hemorrhage. Journal of stroke. 2017;19(1):11-27. doi: 10.5853/jos.2016.00563.

14. Tenny S, Thorell W. Intracranial Hemorrhage..[Updated 2020 Jun 30] In: StatPearls.[Internet] Treasure Island (FL): StatPearls Publishing;; 2020 Jan. Available from: https://www.ncbi.nlm.nih.gov/books/NBK470242/.

15. Graham DI, Adams JH, Nicoll JA, Maxwell WL, Gennarelli TA. The nature, distribution and causes of traumatic brain injury. Brain pathology (Zurich, Switzerland). 1995;5(4):397-406. doi: 10.1111/j.1750-3639.1995.tb00618.x.

16. Haines D, E,. The Meninges. In: Haines DE, Mihailoff GA, editors. Fundamental Neuroscience for Basic and Clinical Applications E-Book. 5th ed.: Elsevier Health Sciences; 2018. p. 107-21.

17. Abraham MK, Chang WW. Subarachnoid Hemorrhage. Emergency medicine clinics of North America. 2016;34(4):901-16. doi: 10.1016/j.emc.2016.06.011.

18. Lederer W, Mair D, Rabl W, Baubin M. Frequency of rib and sternum fractures associated with out-of-hospital cardiopulmonary resuscitation is underestimated by conventional chest X-ray. Resuscitation. 2004;60(2):157-62. doi: 10.1016/j.resuscitation.2003.10.003.

19. Deliliga A, Chatzinikolaou F, Koutsoukis D, Chrysovergis I, Voultsos P. Cardiopulmonary resuscitation (CPR) complications encountered in forensic autopsy cases. BMC emergency medicine. 2019; 19(1):23. doi: 10.1186/s12873-019-0234-5.

20. Baue AE, Blakemore WS. The pericardium. The Annals of thoracic surgery. 1972;14(1):81-106. doi: 10.1016/s0003-4975(10)65204-6.

21. Sutherland I, Ledder O, Crameri J, Nydegger A, Catto-Smith A, Cain T, et al. Pancreatic trauma in children. Pediatric surgery international. 2010;26(12):1201-6. doi: 10.1007/s00383-010-2705-3.

22. Debi U, Kaur R, Prasad KK, Sinha SK, Sinha A, Singh K. Pancreatic trauma: a concise review. World journal of gastroenterology. 2013;19(47):9003-11. doi: 10.3748/wjg.v19.i47.9003.

23. Hussami M, Grabherr S, Meuli RA, Schmidt S. Severe pelvic injury: vascular lesions detected by ante- and post-mortem contrast medium-enhanced CT and associations with pelvic fractures. International journal of legal medicine. 2017;131(3):731-8. doi: 10.1007/s00414-016-1503-4.

24. Makino Y, Yokota H, Hayakawa M, Yajima D, Inokuchi G, Nakatani E, et al. Spinal cord injuries with normal postmortem CT findings: a pitfall of virtual autopsy for detecting traumatic death. AJR American journal of roentgenology. 2014;203(2):240-4. doi: 10.2214/ajr.13.11775.

Chapter 05

Penetrating injuries

5.1. Sharp force

Sharp trauma, such as stab wounds, occurs during homicide, suicide, or accidents. Autopsy investigation of these victims is a component of daily practice in many forensic institutions worldwide, especially those located in countries with high murder rates.[1] The common injury mechanism during sharp trauma is internal damage by the incision of skin, tissue, and organs. The main cause of death is extravasation from injured vessels, which results in hypovolemic shock. However, hemopericardium is also an important cause of death, which causes mechanical restriction of the heartbeat. Air embolism is a newly encountered finding with the introduction of postmortem CT (PMCT) in death investigations, and this finding has frequently been identified as a main cause of death in sharp trauma cases.[2, 3] For the evaluation of stab injuries, forensic questions (e.g., shape, number, location, and channel of wounds, internal organs, and bones involved) should be an-

swered, and the causes of death should be identified. This information is essential for reconstruction of the stabbing incident and excluding the possibility of third-party intervention.[1, 2]

In traditional autopsy examinations, wounds are evaluated by time-consuming dissection of the surrounding tissue layers to determine the direction of the weapon. This method can destroy the trajectory with its surrounding tissue, and thus causes problems in preserving the evidence. Furthermore, abnormal air collection in body cavities or vessels is difficult to identify during the autopsy procedure, and may be impossible after opening those structures.

With the advances in modern CT technologies of multi-detector rows and spiral scanning, radiological images of all possible planes have been obtained through the target structure or lesions in two-dimensional or three-dimensional display modes.[3] PMCT imaging has been incorporated into forensic practices and has shown encouraging results to facilitate answering similar questions posed during the autopsy of sharp trauma cases.[2]

However, regarding superficial injuries of skin and soft tissue, the traditional autopsy procedure continues to yield better results, compared with PMCT.[1] Although an examination of external wounds could be performed by PMCT, such wounds are missed frequently, especially in the event of grouped lesions such as hesitation cuts, mostly due to the limited spatial resolution of current CT scanners.[2] These shortcomings of CT in terms of the detection

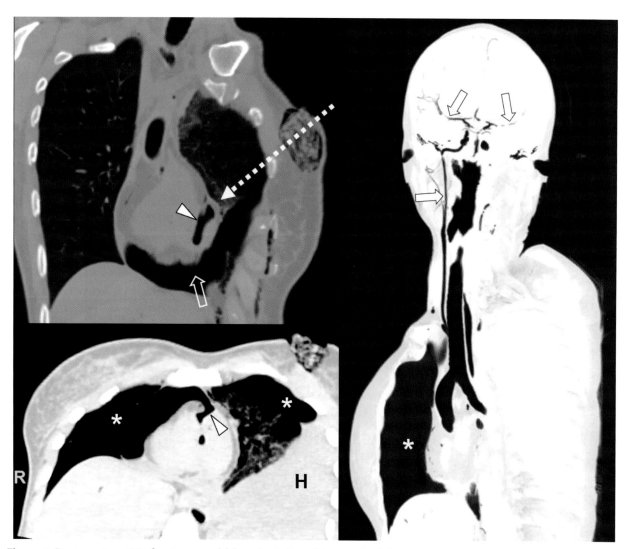

Figure 1. Postmortem CT of a 41-year-old female victim of domestic violence.
Oblique coronal (left upper) image shows an entry site on skin and anterior myocardial defect (arrowhead) of left ventricle, allowing intuitive understanding of blade length and trajectory (dashed arrow). In the oblique axial image (left lower), the heart is displaced by massive hemopneumothorax (H) in the left pleural cavity. The elasticity of the soft tissue and peri- or postmortem changes (e.g., hemorrhage or air collection) may shift the position of the injured site (arrowhead) and organ. Oblique sagittal image (right) shows air embolism in carotid and intracranial arteries. Note massive air collection in the pericardial (arrow) and both pleural cavities (*).

of external or superficial injuries may be complemented by visual inspection in the CT room, in a manner similar to the approach used on the autopsy table.[4] Nevertheless, PMCT imaging should not be used to replace visual inspection of the body surface, but to provide additional information regarding deeper structures.

PMCT can be used to measure the stab channel length accurately, using an appropriate reconstruction plane. However, because of tissue elasticity, the measured channel length can be longer than the length of blade used. Therefore, care should be taken when estimating the size of the weapon involved.[1, 3] PMCT allows for the detection of deeper injuries in various organs (e.g., lungs, heart, liver, and spleen) by showing blood accumulation in the wound channel and in the channel itself. However, regardless of these findings, organ injuries could be clearly presumed by high-density hemorrhage around injured structures (**Fig. 1**).[3, 4]

However, PMCT cannot locate the site of vascular injury and thus cannot differentiate between arterial

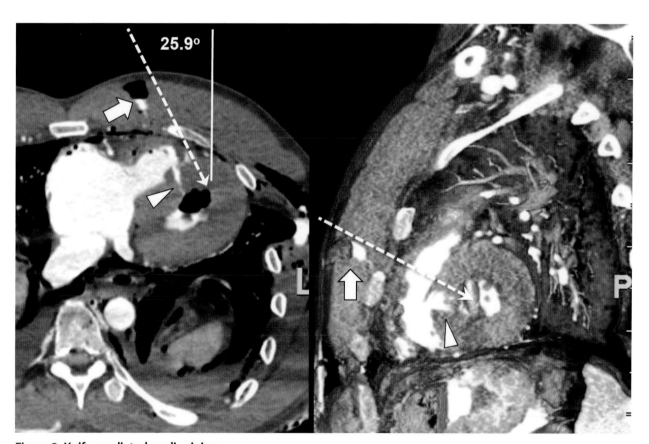

Figure 2. Knife-mediated cardiac injury.
Axial image (right) and three-dimensional oblique sagittal image (left) of postmortem CT angiography in a 48-year-old male show superficial injuries including skin defect and soft tissue hemorrhage (arrows); it also demonstrates deeper myocardial lacerations (arrowheads). In this case, CT was employed to estimate carefully the weapon trajectory and stab channel length, using various image planes in two-dimensional and three-dimensional reconstructions.

and venous bleeding. PMCT angiography (PMCTA) may overcome this limitation of nonenhanced CT by providing a noninvasive representation of the arterial and venous system, as well as by pinpointing the site of vascular damage (**Figs. 2 and 3**).[5, 6]

Recent studies have shown that the vascular lesions found in autopsy examinations are better described by PMCTA, regardless of the cause of vascular damage.[3, 5, 7] Bone lesions are comparatively frequent in cases with sharp trauma and readily found on PMCT. Similar to superficial wounds on visual inspection, skeletal injuries found on CT can provide hints regarding the type of weapon involved; they can also guide autopsy dissection for the careful exposure of lesions to add visual analysis to the digital information.[1, 2] For the investigation of the cause of death, PMCT has been proven very useful. According to a study.[2] of sharp traumatic injuries, PMCT could be used to find or suggest nearly all relevant findings described at the autopsy in relation to potential causes of death. Their results revealed that PMCT is useful to assess fatal injuries (e.g., massive extravasation, hemo-

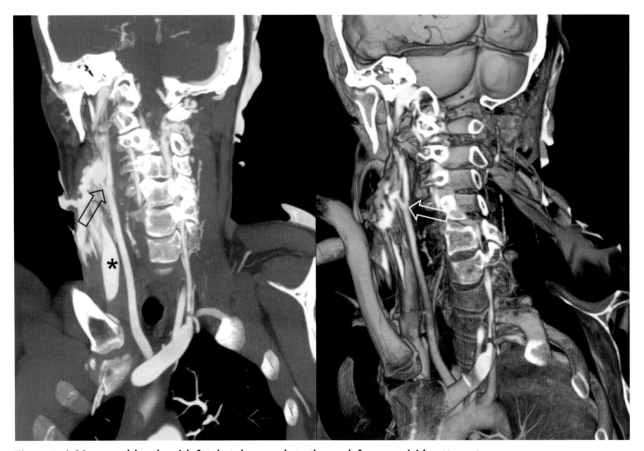

Figure 3. A 29-year-old male with fatal stab wounds to the neck from a suicide attempt.
Coronal maximum intensity projection image (left) and three-dimensional volume-rendered image (right) of postmortem CT angiography clearly depict the knife trajectory and localize the site of vascular injury, showing the point of external carotid artery severing (arrow) and soft tissue injury (*).

pericardium, or pneumothorax) in all cases of stab fatalities. In addition, PMCT suggested air embolism as a potential cause of death, which would be difficult or sometimes impossible to be identified when using conventional autopsy techniques.[3] The superiority of PMCT has been clearly demonstrated with regard to the description of abnormal air collection in the body, including subcutaneous emphysema, pneumothorax, and air embolism.[8-10] (**Fig. 4 and 5**).

However, in our experience, these findings are unlikely to be found in the conventional autopsy unless informed or suspected in advance. The presence of venous air embolism can be explained by the entry of external air through damaged walls while the injured person remains alive and blood flow persists.[4] Occasionally, the systemic vascular bed is filled with air. In those situations, air must have entered the arterial system through stab-induced arteriovenous shunts, if the victim does not have an open foramen ovale or ductus arteriosus.[2] Massive air embolism itself is a fatal condition that may lead to death. In those cases, the mechanism of death is generally regarded as right heart failure caused by sudden mechanical blockage of the pulmonary arterial system and subsequent elevation of right ventricular pressure, as observed in cases of massive pulmonary thromboembolism.[11, 12] In cases of cerebral air embolism, air bubbles can occlude the vascular lumen and block blood flow to the brain parenchyma, resulting in hypoxic brain damage and death.[11-13] However, because the origins of air in blood vessels vary, care is needed when interpreting gases in the vascular system as air embolism.[4, 10]

Generally, the distribution pattern of gas in the body helps to differentiate air embolism reliably from putrefaction (i.e., the most common source of gas). Gas collection limited to the right heart and vascular system is a finding indicative of air embolism. In contrast, the intestinal wall and mesenteric and portal venous systems are the first sites of putrefactive gas on PMCT, followed by right heart chambers and then other sites in the body.[14] Three-dimensional reconstruction of CT images is a useful technique to diagnose air embolism in cases with fatal stab injuries, by reliably demonstrating the amount and distribution of the gas in the cardiac chambers and blood vessels.[3] Cardiopulmonary resuscitation (CPR) is another potential source of intravascular air. Air may be forced into the circulatory system via ruptured pulmonary vessels during intense CPR.[15] Therefore, after vigorous resuscitation, it is difficult to determine whether air in blood vessels is due to air embolism associated with stab wounds or solely a perimortem artifact related to CPR.

In cases involving an atypical weapon, PMCT can be used to determine the injury mechanism by estimating the force direction, weapon penetration depth, and bony fragment pattern (**Fig. 6**).

In summary, although there remain limitations with respect to thorough external examinations, PMCT may be useful for evaluating fatal cases with sharp trauma. In addition to the detection of bone injuries and air embolism, PMCT may guide autopsy planning and facilitate tailored dissection to increase the overall likelihood of identifying traumatic injuries without evidence destruction. This is particularly true of the investigation of vessel injuries with PMCTA.

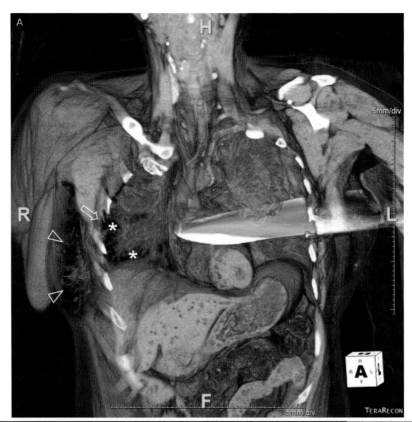

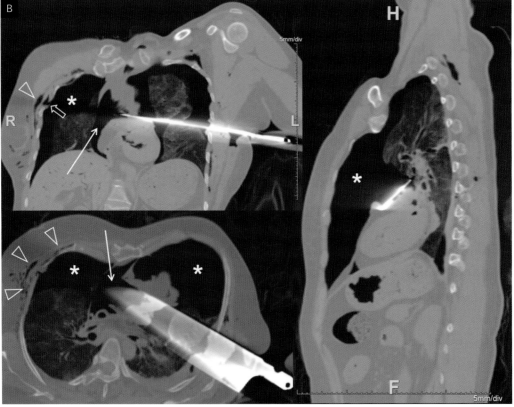

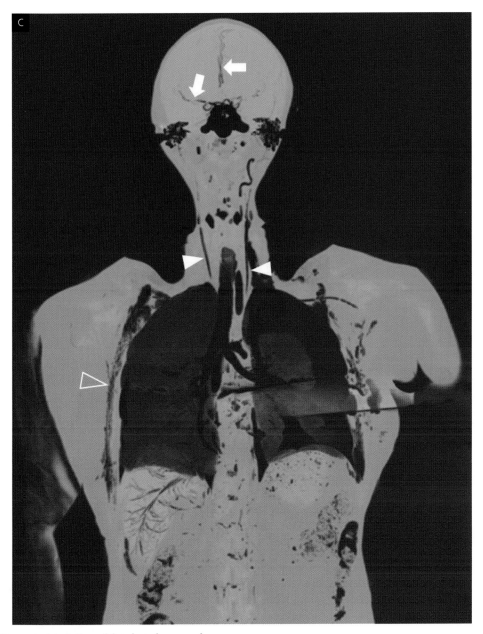

Figure 4. A 58-year-old victim of fatal stab wound.
(A) Three-dimensional volume-rendered image. (B) Multiplanar reformation oblique coronal (left upper), oblique axial (left lower), and sagittal (right) images. (C) Minimum intensity projection (MinIP) image. (A, B) Postmortem CT shows a knife in the victim's body, aiding in estimation of the penetration distance and direction of the weapon without autopsy photographs. In addition to pneumothorax (*) and pneumopericardium (long arrows), CT depicts contralateral pleural and chest wall injury (arrow) with soft tissue emphysema (arrowheads) and facilitates estimation of the maximum penetration depth of the knife (i.e., passing through both lungs and reaching the opposite chest wall). Note the presence of soft tissue emphysema on the chest wall, which provides evidence of vitality immediately after stabbing (A-C). (C) MinIP image shows air collection in both internal carotid arteries (white arrowheads) and cerebral arteries (white arrows), corresponding to systemic air embolism as well as chest wall emphysema (arrowhead). Unless there are open congenital intracardiac (i.e., patent foramen ovale or septal defects) or extracardiac shunts (i.e., patent ductus arteriosus or pulmonary shunt), this gas presumably entered the systemic vascular bed via stab-induced arteriovenous shunts.

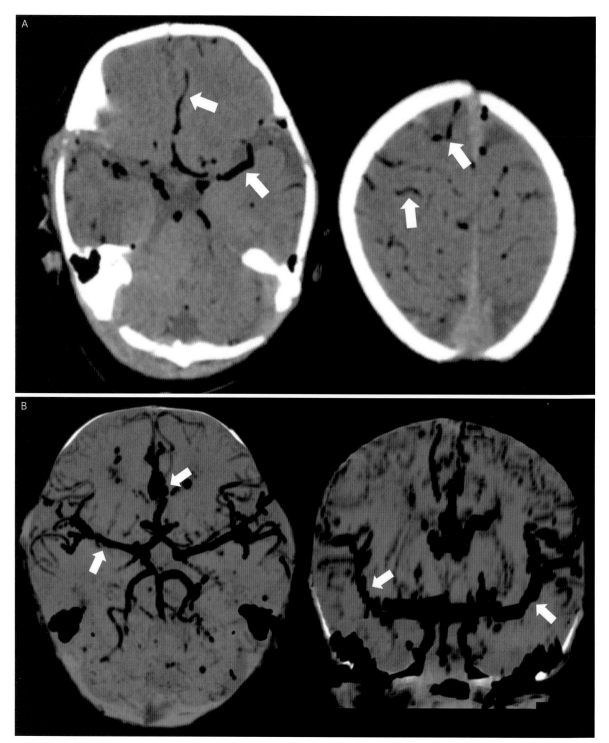

Figure 5. Postmortem CT of a 6-day-old male who received vigorous and prolonged cardiopulmonary resuscitation.
The patient exhibited cardiac arrest during intravenous sampling and fluid therapy for rotavirus infection. Minimal intensity projection thin-slab axial images (A) and thick slab axial and coronal images (B) show extensive air collection in cerebral arteries (arrows), corresponding to massive systemic air embolism after vigorous and prolonged cardiopulmonary resuscitation.

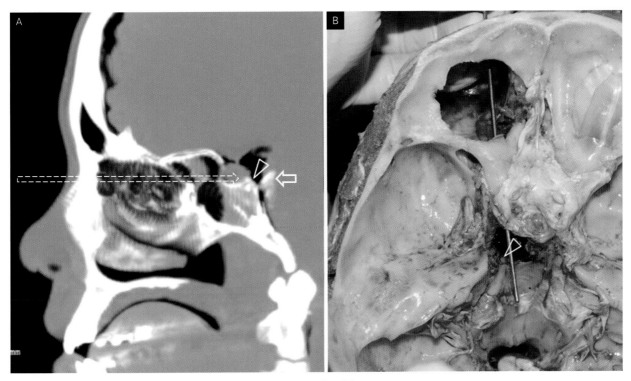

Figure 6. A case of a penetrating brain injury through the orbital fossa.
Coronal image from postmortem CT (A) shows brainstem injury by bone fragments (arrow) from the dorsum sellae (arrowhead), which was presumably fractured by the tip of the sharp object that entered the victim's eye. CT estimated the direction (dotted arrow) and penetration depth of the weapon, thus aiding in establishment of the injury mechanism, which was later confirmed in autopsy dissection (B). Note the presence of fracture of the dorsum sellae (arrowhead) and pathway of the weapon (tip of an umbrella) through the orbital fossa to the cranial cavity. The frontal bone was partially removed to show the potential course of the weapon (represented by a metallic wire).

References

1   Woźniak KJ, Moskała A, Grabherr S. Sharp Trauma. In: Grabherr S, Grimm JM, Heinemann A, editors. Atlas of Postmortem Angiography. Cham: Springer International Publishing; 2016. p. 411-51.

2   Schnider J, Thali MJ, Ross S, Oesterhelweg L, Spendlove D, Bolliger SA. Injuries due to sharp trauma detected by post-mortem multislice computed tomography (MSCT): a feasibility study. Legal medicine (Tokyo, Japan). 2009;11(1):4-9. doi: 10.1016/j.legalmed.2008.07.001.

3   Lee H, Lee S, Cha JG, Baek T, Yang KM. Postmortem Computed Tomography and Computed Tomography Angiography: Cardiothoracic Imaging Applications in Forensic Medicine. Journal of thoracic imaging. 2019;34(5):286-98. doi: 10.1097/rti.0000000000000398.

4   Zerbini T, Silva LF, Ferro AC, Kay FU, Amaro Junior E, Pasqualucci CA, et al. Differences between postmortem computed tomography and conventional autopsy in a stabbing murder case. Clinics (Sao Paulo, Brazil). 2014;69(10):683-7. doi: 10.6061/clinics/2014(10)06.

5   Ross S, Spendlove D, Bolliger S, Christe A, Oesterhelweg L, Grabherr S, et al. Postmortem whole-body CT angiography: evaluation of two contrast media solutions. AJR American journal of roentgenology. 2008;190(5):1380-9. doi: 10.2214/ajr.07.3082.

6   Jackowski C, Sonnenschein M, Thali MJ, Aghayev E, von Allmen G, Yen K, et al. Virtopsy: postmortem minimally invasive angiography using cross section techniques--implementation and preliminary results. Journal of forensic sciences. 2005;50(5):1175-86.

7   Grabherr S, Grimm J, Dominguez A, Vanhaebost J, Mangin P. Advances in post-mortem CT-angiography. The British journal of radiology. 2014;87(1036):20130488. doi: 10.1259/bjr.20130488.

8   Cha JG, Kim DH, Kim DH, Paik SH, Park JS, Park SJ, et al. Utility of postmortem autopsy via whole-body imaging: initial observations comparing MDCT and 3.0 T MRI findings with autopsy findings. Korean journal of radiology. 2010;11(4):395-406. doi: 10.3348/kjr.2010.11.4.395.

9   Thali MJ, Yen K, Schweitzer W, Vock P, Boesch C, Ozdoba C, et al. Virtopsy, a new imaging horizon in forensic pathology: virtual autopsy by postmortem multislice computed tomography (MSCT) and magnetic resonance imaging (MRI)--a feasibility study. Journal of forensic sciences. 2003;48(2):386-403.

10 Ali Z, Bolster F, Goldberg E, Fowler D, Li L. Systemic air embolism complicating upper gastrointestinal endoscopy: a case report with post-mortem CT scan findings and review of literature. Forensic sciences research. 2016;1(1):52-7. doi: 10.1080/20961790.2016.1252898.

11 Lee H. Massive Intraventricular Air Embolism after Contrast-enhanced CT: Report of Two Cases. J Korean Radiol Soc. 2006;54:349-52.

12 Rahman ZU, Murtaza G, Pourmorteza M, El Minaoui WK, Sethi P, Mamdouhi P, et al. Cardiac Arrest as a Consequence of Air Embolism: A Case Report and Literature Review. Case reports in medicine. 2016;2016:8236845. doi: 10.1155/2016/8236845.

13 Andenmatten MA, Thali MJ, Kneubuehl BP, Oesterhelweg L, Ross S, Spendlove D, et al. Gunshot injuries detected by post-mortem multislice computed tomography (MSCT): a feasibility study. Legal medicine (Tokyo, Japan). 2008;10(6):287-92. doi: 10.1016/j.legalmed.2008.03.005.

14 Egger C, Bize P, Vaucher P, Mosimann P, Schneider B, Dominguez A, et al. Distribution of artifactual gas on post-mortem multidetector computed tomography (MDCT). International journal of legal medicine. 2012;126(1):3-12. doi: 10.1007/s00414-010-0542-5.

15 Hwang SL, Lieu AS, Lin CL, Liu GC, Howng SL, Kuo TH. Massive cerebral air embolism after cardiopulmonary resuscitation. Journal of clinical neuroscience : official journal of the Neurosurgical Society of Australasia. 2005;12(4):468-9. doi: 10.1016/j.jocn.2004.03.041.

5.2. Gunshot wound—Entry, trajectory, and foreign bodies

General characteristics of gunshot wounds are the presence of soft tissue damage in the entry site, along with contusion hematoma (i.e., bruises) around the entry wound.[1] In cases of close-range shootings, a typical "gunpowder tattoo" can be observed at the wound site, which is characterized by the presence of gunpowder particles lodged in burned skin (stippling) by hot exhaust gases from the gun muzzle.[1, 2] The primary questions that should be addressed in the evaluation of gunshot injuries include the location of entry and exit wounds, firing distance, presence of bullets and their fragments in the body, trajectories of bullets, related tissue and organ injuries, and causes of death.[2] However, these features may not be evident when evaluating severely decomposed bodies.[1]

PMCT has been widely used for the evaluation of firearm fatalities in many forensic centers worldwide. CT imaging is reportedly a successful adjuvant to traditional autopsy for detecting the entry and exit wounds, internal or external beveling of bones, bullets and fragments in the body, trajectory and direction of firing, and firing range (**Fig. 1**).

Furthermore, PMCT is comparable to autopsy for detecting the cause of death in cases of gunshot injuries. The causes of death described by PMCT are reportedly consistent with the causes diagnosed by autopsy. Moreover, CT reportedly detects more injuries and abnormalities than autopsy in various body structures and organs (e.g., abnormal air collection).[3, 4]

In gunshot fatalities to the head, CT can be a useful tool to demonstrate head injuries. One study showed that PMCT could identify entry and exit wounds in nearly all cases with craniocerebral injuries.[5] PMCT also has been proven useful for assessing the bullet path in the brain because it can reveal the bullet trajectory by depicting patterns of bone fragments or hemorrhage through the brain parenchyma, or by connecting entry and exit wounds. However, it is challenging to evaluate gunshot wounds elsewhere in the body. In a study regarding the role of CT in evaluation of gunshot casualties, PMCT helped to identify entry wounds in 69.2% of cases and exit wounds in 52.2% of cases; it determined the bullet trajectory in 72.1% of penetrating wounds throughout the body. In cases with multiple shots, it is more challenging to evaluate each bullet's trajectory when several projectiles are close to each other or multiple external wounds exist.[3, 6] Furthermore, PMCT imaging has minimal effectiveness in identifying injuries to solid organs, such as the liver, spleen, and diaphragm. Although CT can show hemorrhage in solid organs and body cavities, it cannot specify the exact locations of organ damages or major vascular lacerations, whereas these aspects can be directly explored by visual inspection during autopsy. In most cases with solid organ injuries or multiple hits, autopsy is reportedly better for detecting external wounds, wound channels, trajectories, and organ injuries. Similarly, the CT diagnosis of hollow viscus perforation is established mostly on the basis of the presence of free air without specifying the perforation site.[6] This is presumably because of the low contrast resolution of nonenhanced CT, compared with the

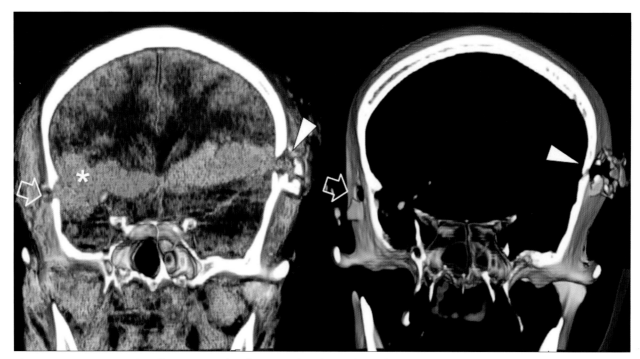

Figure 1. Postmortem CT of a young male who committed suicide with a gun.
Three-dimensional volume-rendered coronal image with soft tissue (left) and bone (right) setting. A bullet entered the right temporal area and exited from the left temporal area. Coronal image with soft tissue setting shows that the wound channel is filled with hemorrhage. Note the presence of internal and external beveling of bones, each characteristic of entry and exit wounds. Bone setting image shows a rounded and fairly well circumscribed bony defect at the entry wound and multiple bony fragments bursting out of the exit wound.

resolution that can be achieved with the naked eye.[3] However, with the introduction of angiography techniques into the postmortem setting, CT imaging is reportedly comparable to autopsy for the detection of organ damage, and may be better for the precise localization of vascular rupture.[7]

In the evaluation of skeletal injuries, PMCT is particularly useful for the visualization of subtle fractures and bony fragments, which can easily be missed in a visual inspection (**Fig. 2**).

Three-dimensional reconstruction of image data provides an overview of skeletal fractures and dis-

placement, which could offer clues to explain injury mechanisms. PMCT was superior to autopsy for the detection of fractures in the cranial vault, facial bones, ribs, vertebral bodies, and pelvic bones.[3, 8] Some of these fractures are not easily accessible and thus are time-consuming to explore during autopsy.

PMCT has a distinct advantage in ballistic interpretation involving the detection of foreign objects. This detection is a primary aspect of PMCT imaging. Many studies have reported that PMCT is an excellent tool for the detection and localization of retained bullets and their fragments before opening the body,

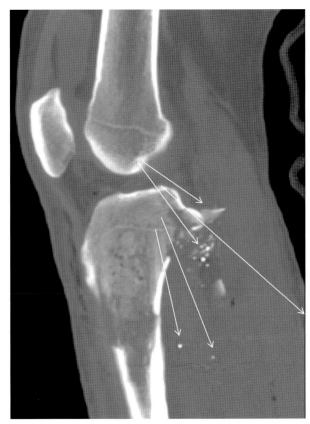

Figure 2. Gunshot damage to the knee.
Sagittal image of postmortem CT shows the destruction of tibia with the distribution pattern of bone fragments, revealing the direction of injury and trajectory of the bullet in the body.

especially in the context of advanced decomposition. Therefore, PMCT can guide the effective removal of foreign bodies and evaluation of surrounding tissue damage in an autopsy (**Fig. 3**).

Another obvious advantage of PMCT is its ability to detect air collection in various body structures in cases of air embolism. PMCT is reportedly simple and more reliable than autopsy for the detection of abnormal air accumulations (e.g., air embolism, pneumothorax, and pneumoperitoneum), which are

usually not detected through the conventional autopsy procedure unless specialized dissection methods or tools are used.[2] Currently, PMCT is the sole tool widely used in many forensic institutions worldwide to detect abnormal air collection in the context of routine autopsies.[7]

Another important forensic question that should be addressed is the firing distance. In cases of close or intermediate range shots (approximately <30 inches or 76 cm), CT allows the detection of gunshot residue (stippling or tattooing by unburned bullet powder) around the entry wound. However, the assessment of firing range is mainly based on visual examination of wound shape and adjacent skin changes, as well as the chemical detection of gunshot residues and their distribution around the entrance wound.

In summary, CT is a useful tool to complement the postmortem investigation of gunshot fatalities. It enables the detection and precise positional location of bullets and their fragments, as well as associated injuries, in structures that are difficult to approach during routine autopsies. PMCT can also be used to determine the causes of death, in a manner consistent with the causes determined by autopsy in most cases. In cases of multiple gunshots, autopsy is superior for the detection of entry wounds, injury direction, and wound channels. However, imaging is reportedly better than autopsy for the detection of bony fractures, foreign bodies, and abnormal air collection (e.g., air embolism and pneumothorax)[3], which might escape observation during routine autopsies.

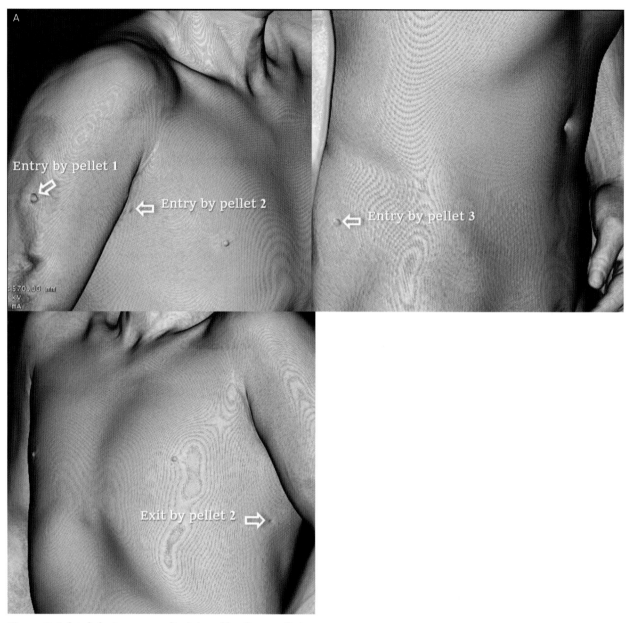

Figure 3. A fatal shotgun casualty injured by three pellets.
Postmortem CT shows one (pellet 2) completely perforated and two (pellet 1 and 3) remaining in the body. Note the presence of three entry wounds and one exit wound (A) with their trajectories (B-E). In this case, PMCT allowed identification of the bullet locations near the spinous process of thoracic spine (pellet 1 in C) and sacrum (pellet 3 in E); these areas are difficult to explore during autopsy. PMCT also demonstrated the presence of pneumothorax (*) and related soft tissue emphysema (short arrows) in the lateral chest wall, as well as hemopericardium (HP) and massive bilateral hemothorax (HT). In this case, the findings of pneumothorax and soft tissue emphysema serve as a vital sign (i.e., evidence of vitality) in the victim at the time of shooting (C, D). These findings help estimate the trajectory of bullets in the body by drawing lines between the entry and exit wounds (d) and the bullets in the body (C, E).
a, b: Three-dimensional volume-rendered images; c: axial (upper), coronal (lower left), and sagittal (lower right) images; d: axial (upper) and coronal (lower) images; e: axial (upper), coronal (lower left), and sagittal (lower right) images.

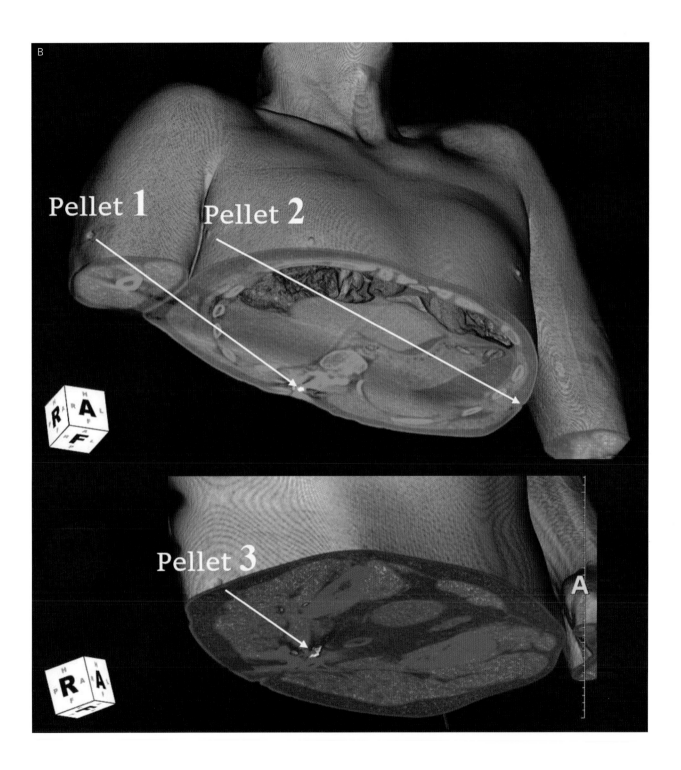

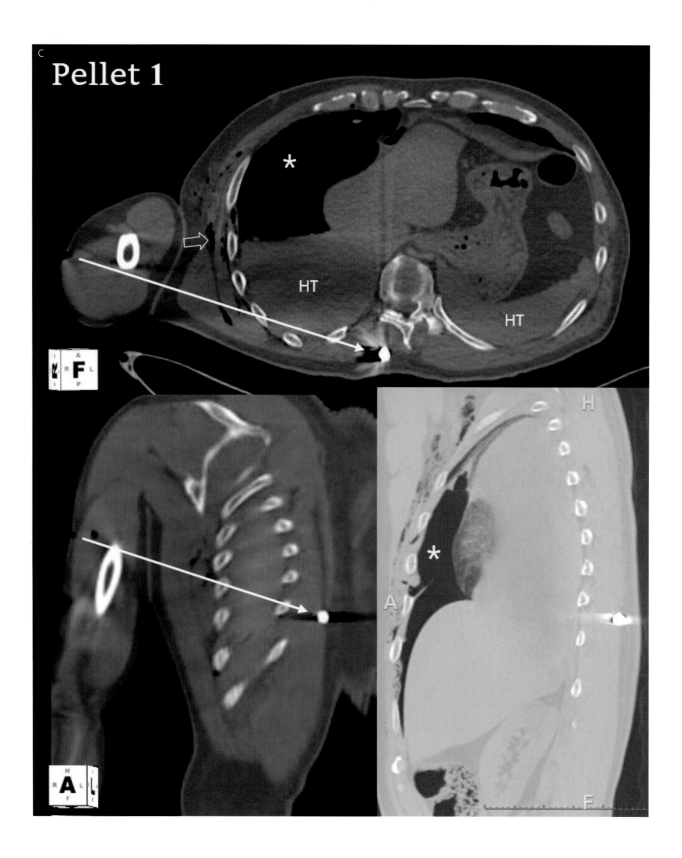

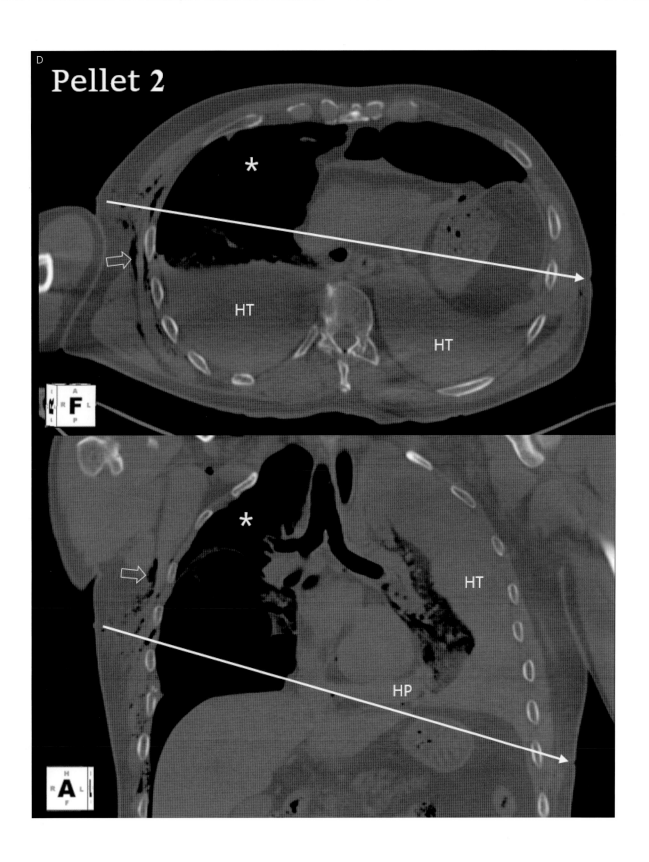

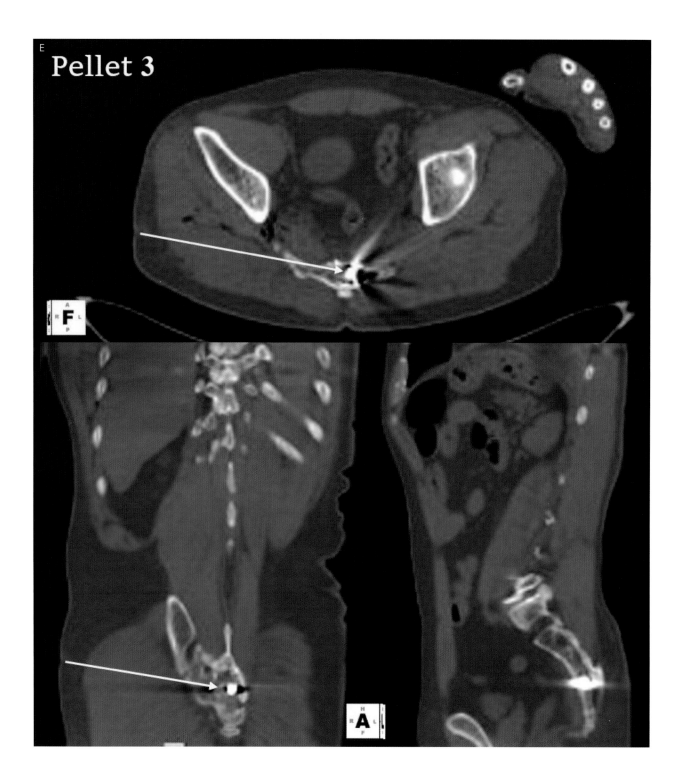

Pellet 3

References

1   Wojciechowski A, Fudalej M, Skowronek P. Assessment of head gunshot wounds by means of post-mortem computed tomography in exhumed anonymous cadaver. BJR case reports. 2016;2(4): 20150304. doi: 10.1259/bjrcr.20150304.

2   Andenmatten MA, Thali MJ, Kneubuehl BP, Oesterhelweg L, Ross S, Spendlove D, et al. Gunshot injuries detected by post-mortem multislice computed tomography (MSCT): a feasibility study. Legal medicine (Tokyo, Japan). 2008;10(6):287-92. doi: 10.1016/j. legalmed. 2008.03.005.

3   Elkhateeb SA, Mohammed EB, Meleka HA, Ismail AAE. Postmortem computed tomography and autopsy for detection of lesions and causes of death in gunshot injury cases: a comparative study. Egyptian Journal of Forensic Sciences. 2018;8(1):50. doi: 10.1186/s41935-018-0078-2.

4   Lathrop SL, Nolt eKB. Utility of Postmortem X-ray Computed Tomography (CT) in Supplanting or Supplementing Medicolegal Autopsies. National Institute of Justice; 2015.

5   Oehmichen M, Meissner C, König HG, Gehl HB. Gunshot injuries to the head and brain caused by low-velocity handguns and rifles. A review. Forensic science international. 2004;146(2-3):111-20. doi: 10.1016/j.forsciint.2004.06.023.

6   Makhlouf F, Scolan V, Ferretti G, Stahl C, Paysant F. Gunshot fatalities: correlation between post-mortem multi-slice computed tomography and autopsy findings: a 30-months retrospective study. Legal medicine (Tokyo, Japan). 2013;15(3):145-8. doi: 10.1016/j.legalmed. 2012.11.002.

7   Lee H, Lee S, Cha JG, Baek T, Yang KM. Postmortem Computed Tomography and Computed Tomography Angiography: Cardiothoracic Imaging Applications in Forensic Medicine. Journal of thoracic imaging. 2019;34(5):286-98. doi: 10.1097/rti.0000000000000398.

8   Poulsen K, Simonsen J. Computed tomography as routine in connection with medico-legal autopsies. Forensic science international. 2007;171(2-3):190-7. doi: 10.1016/j.forsciint.2006.05.041.

Chapter 06

Blast injury

Explosions can create distinctive injury patterns that are difficult to identify outside of battle, causing life-threatening multi-organ injuries in many people simultaneously.[1] The basic mechanism of explosion damage involves the conversion of a solid or liquid into a rapidly expanding gas, creating a high-pressure blast wave that traverses bodies and objects, followed by a high-speed blast wind that produces flying debris from explosive devices or surroundings (Fig. 1).[2]

Explosions produce a blast wave which consist of a shock wave and a blast wind.[3, 4] A shock wave refers to the initial spike of high positive air pressure (i.e., wave front, shock front, or blast wave in a narrow sense) that expands supersonically.[3] and radially from an explosive source, lasting for a few milliseconds.[4, 5] This rapid increase in pressure (i.e., over-pressurization) is caused by compression of the atmosphere that comprises the wave front from an explosion.[3-6] The blast wind is a flow of superheated air behind the initial shock wave,

which is produced by the mass movement of air due to the rapid expansion of explosion gases.[5] Initially, it travels outward from the explosion core[4], interacting with victims and causing damage.[7] Continuous expansion of air leads to an immediate negative-pressure phase (i.e., under-pressurization below normal atmospheric pressure) the tail of the blast wave[3], and the blast wind reverses its direction and blows back toward the explosion core.[3, 6] A victim close to the explosion will encounter both the high-pressure shock wave and the subsequent high-speed wind.[3] Explosives are classified as high-order or low-order: a high-order explosive creates a high-pressure shock wave that propagates supersonically, while a low-order explosive produces a subsonic explosion without a shock wave.[7] Importantly, a blast wind can be caused by either high-order or low-order explosives.[1, 4]

In general, blast injuries are classified into four distinct mechanisms that occur sequentially (Fig. 1). Death can result from one or more of these mecha-

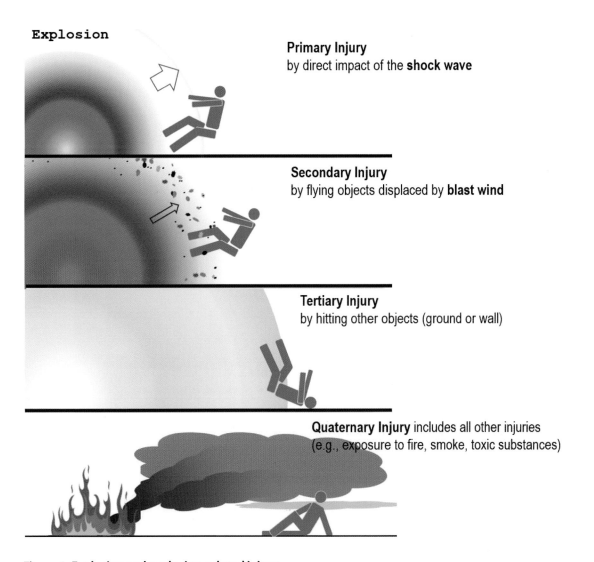

Explosion

Primary Injury
by direct impact of the **shock wave**

Secondary Injury
by flying objects displaced by **blast wind**

Tertiary Injury
by hitting other objects (ground or wall)

Quaternary Injury includes all other injuries
(e.g., exposure to fire, smoke, toxic substances)

Figure 1. Explosion and explosion-related injury.
Explosion is defined as the sudden release of energy by an extensive compression of surrounding medium and subsequent increase in pressure. In the event of surface explosion, the resulting overpressure wave (i.e., blast wave) propagates as a sphere of compressed air and is immediately followed by a negative-pressure wave due to the overexpansion of air. A blast wave has a shock wave comprising the initial pulse of strong positive air pressure produced by an explosion, which expands supersonically from the core*. The blast wind, the later part of a blast wave, is a mass of rapidly moving air behind the shock wave. Initially, it travels outward from the explosion core; its direction is later reversed during the negative phase of the blast wave. Blast injuries comprise four distinct mechanisms; blast wave impact on the body (primary), various flying debris displaced by the blast wind (secondary), body impact on the surface of the ground or wall due to the blast wind (tertiary), or other explosion-related injuries that are not caused by the first three mechanisms (quaternary).

* Currently, the term blast wave is also used to refer only to the initial shock wave in a narrow sense.

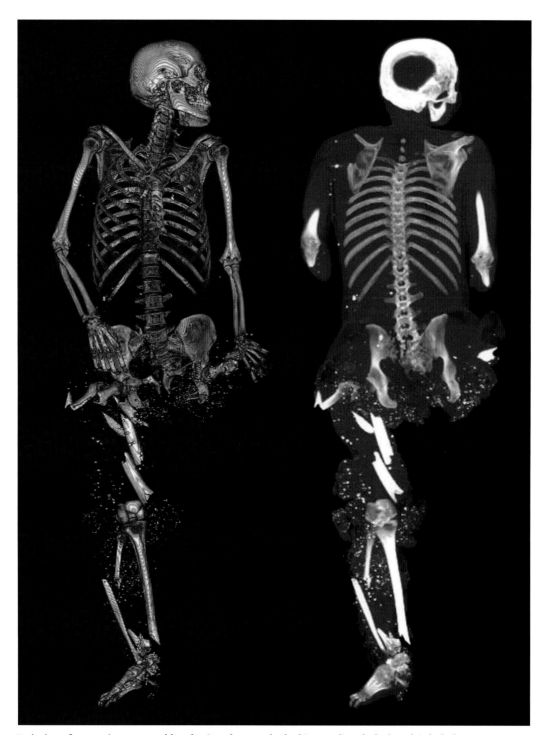

Figure 2. A victim of an anti-personnel land mine that exploded immediately below his left foot.

Whole-body PMCT images show that the victim's left lower extremity was blown off by the shock wave at the level of the hip joint. Moreover, the right side was completely destroyed with multiple bone fractures, acetabular dislocation, and extensive soft tissue loss. Note the presence of multiple fragments and shrapnel distributed throughout the body, particularly in the lower half of the body. Three-dimensional volume rendered image (left) and Maximum intensity projection (right).

nisms. Injury patterns depend on multiple factors including the type and strength of explosion, environment of the blast (closed vs. open space), and the distance of the victim from the explosion.

Primary blast injury is caused by direct impact of the high-pressure shock front (blast wave) on the body surface and its transmission through the body. The effect of this overpressure wave results in extensive damage to air-containing organs (e.g., lungs, ears, eyes, and portions of the gastrointestinal tract), regardless of external injuries.[4] Blast lung injuries (e.g., pulmonary contusion, edema, and barotrauma-related hemorrhage) are the most common fatal primary injury and most common cause of death among the initial survivors of an explosion.[1, 4] However, injuries to brain and abdominal solid organs can occur; these include brain hemorrhage, blast-induced neurotrauma (e.g., cognitive deficits, brain edema, diffuse axonal damage, and long-term neurological deficits) and rupture of the liver, spleen, and kidneys.[4] In addition, generalized injuries that cause instant death (e.g., full body disruption, generalized damage to the body without disintegration, and amputations of the extremities) can be caused by blast overpressure for victims in close proximity to the explosion core **(Fig. 2)**.[2] Because only high-order explosives generate a shock wave, this type of injury is specific to high-order explosions.[7]

Secondary blast injury results from the propulsion of projectiles by the explosion blast wind.[1, 2, 4, 7] The projectiles originate from either the bomb itself (bomb fragments and shrapnel).[4] or local materials around the explosion. Secondary blast injuries are more common than primary injuries and contribute to most casualties among victims of many explosions. The resulting injuries are either penetrating or blunt-traumatic, including various injuries to the skin, soft tissue, internal organs, or bony structures (e.g., abrasion, lacerations, hematomas, and fractures). Occasionally, fatal injuries occur when flying particles penetrate vital organs, such as the brain and heart. Anti-personnel bombs or landmines for conventional military action are explosives specifically designed to inflict more injuries by flying shrapnel and bomb fragments **(Fig. 3)**. In homemade or improvised explosives for terrorist attacks, however, various objects (e.g., nails, screws, bearings, and bolts) are often placed around or embedded into the bombs to injure large numbers of individuals.[7]

Tertiary injuries occur when an individual is thrown by the blast wind and hits other objects, or when a structure collapses and crushes an individual's body.[4, 7] This results in common blunt injuries such as fractures, amputations, internal hemorrhage, and head injuries. Penetrating injury may occur if the victim is thrown against sharp objects. Quaternary injuries comprise any physical and psychological injuries not included in the first three injury categories. These injuries result from exposure to fire, smoke, chemical substances (e.g., sarin and other toxic gases), radiation (e.g., from dirty bombs), and biological agents (e.g., anthrax).[4] After-explosion psychological impacts include severe anxiety, depression, and flashbacks that can lead to post-traumatic stress disorder.[7, 8]

In the clinical setting, CT plays an important role as the primary imaging modality used to assess blast injuries and triage patients for surgical intervention.[9]

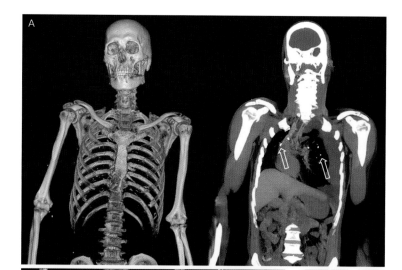

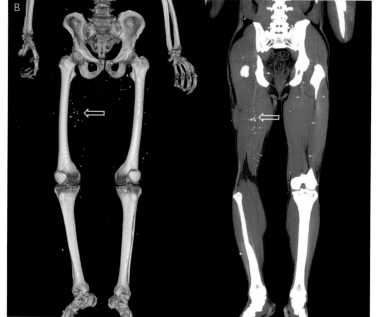

Figure 3. A victim of an anti-personnel land mine that exploded at close range.

Three-dimensional volume-rendered image (left) and maximum intensity projection image (right) in both (A) and (B). Multiplanar reformatted images in parasagittal (left) and axial planes (right) in (C).

In this case, visual inspections showed no apparent injuries on the skin, but revealed small penetrating wounds throughout the body. Postmortem CT images show penetration of the shrapnel and bomb fragments into the superficial soft tissues, muscles, chest wall, and lungs (arrows in a and B). Postmortem CT also revealed multiple projectiles located deep in the cerebellum (arrowheads in C), which might have resulted in instant death for this victim. These particles, along with particles in the soft tissue of the neck, were distributed in such a manner that the trajectory of the projectiles (dotted arrow) and stance of body posture at the time of the explosion could be postulated. Secondary explosive injuries are generally obvious and may be small on the external surface of the body. However, the consequences can be deceptive and more devastating than they appear on the skin, because bomb particles and debris on the ground are propelled several times faster than bullets. This case clearly illustrates a small surface wound hiding a fatal injury underneath it.

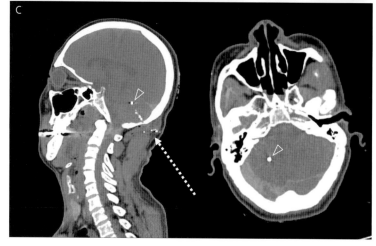

In cases of penetrating injuries, CT is useful for the detection and positional location of foreign bodies (e.g., shrapnel or debris from surroundings), thus providing images from various postprocessing methods in all possible planes. CT angiography is performed to determine the presence and location of vascular injuries in affected body regions. In the postmortem setting, CT is a useful imaging tool for determining the cause of death through the detection of foreign bodies and their trajectories, which can cause fatal internal injuries. In addition, three-dimensional image reconstructions provide pictorial representations of complex injuries and may facilitate an intuitive understanding of the injury pattern, particularly in cases with a combination of distinct blast injury mechanisms.

References

1   Centers for Disease Control and Prevention. Explosions and Blast Injuries: A Primer for Clinicians. 2013.

2   Barrios MZ, Rúa FJC, Restrepo R. Description of blast injuries: literature review, case report and proposal for a new classification. Case Reports. 2015;1:60-76.

3   Cullis IG. Blast waves and how they interact with structures. Journal of the Royal Army Medical Corps. 2001;147(1):16-26. doi: 10.1136/jramc-147-01-02.

4   Born CT. Blast trauma: the fourth weapon of mass destruction. Scandinavian journal of surgery : SJS : official organ for the Finnish Surgical Society and the Scandinavian Surgical Society. 2005;94(4): 279-85. doi: 10.1177/145749690509400406.

5   Institute of Medicine. Pathophysiology of Blast Injury and Overview of Experimental Data. Gulf War and Health: Volume 9: Long-Term Effects of Blast Exposures. Washington, DC: The National Academies Press; 2014. p. 33-83.

6   Departments of the Army tN, and the Air force,. Effects of nuclear explosions. NATO handbook on the medical aspects of NBC depensive operations AMedP-6(B) part I - nuclear. 1996. p. 5-8.

7   Jorolemon M, Lopez R, Krywko D. Blast Injuries. [Updated 2020 Jul 19] StatPearls.[Internet] Treasure Island (FL): StatPearls Publishing; 2020-Jan.

8   Elder GA, Dorr NP, De Gasperi R, Gama Sosa MA, Shaughness MC, Maudlin-Jeronimo E, et al. Blast exposure induces post-traumatic stress disorder-related traits in a rat model of mild traumatic brain injury. Journal of neurotrauma. 2012;29(16):2564-75. doi: 10.1089/neu.2012.2510.

9   Yazgan C, Aksu NM. Imaging features of blast injuries: experience from 2015 Ankara bombing in Turkey. The British journal of radiology. 2016;89(1062):20160063. doi: 10.1259/bjr.20160063.

Death
by asphyxiation

Chapter 07

Strangulation

The term "strangulation" refers to a form of asphyxia that involves obstruction of air passage to the lungs and blood flow to the brain, due to external compression of the neck.[1-3] Strangulation is further divided into three categories: hanging, ligature strangulation, and manual strangulation, based on the origin of constricting pressure. Specifically, hanging involves the use of any material around the neck, tightened by the gravitational weight of the strangled body; ligature strangulation involves the use of any material around the neck, tightened by a force other than body weight; and manual strangulation

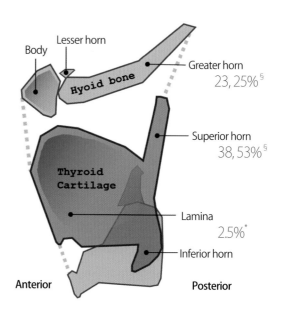

Figure 1. Lateral anatomy of hyoid-larynx complex and frequency of thyroid skeleton injuries in suicidal hanging.
§ from References 5 and 6.
* Lamina and inferior horn injury, from Reference 6.

involves compression pressure from the offender's hands, forearms, or knees.[2, 3] Regardless of the subtype of strangulation, in cases of fatalities, the cause of death is presumably cerebral hypoxia due to the compression of blood vessels.[2, 3]

Practically, hanging is defined as the suspension of a person by a ligature around the neck. It can be further classified as either complete hanging with free suspension of the body above the ground, or incomplete (partial) hanging with parts of the body touching the ground and supporting the victim's weight.[2] The term "near hanging" refers to individuals who survive a hanging for a sufficient duration to reach the hospital. In the visual inspection of hanging cases, ligature marks and underlying subcutaneous desiccation may be the pathognomonic signs; without these, hanging can be excluded as a mechanism of neck trauma and death.[4] The desiccation refers to dehydrated thinning of soft tissue due to the extrusion of tissue fluid by mechanical compression.

Other relevant findings in hanging cases include soft tissue hemorrhage (subcutaneous and intramuscular) and fractures of the throat skeleton (**Fig. 1**). The most common injury found during autopsy of suicidal hangings is hematoma in the sternocleidomastoid muscle, followed by fracture of the superior horn of the thyroid cartilage and greater horn of the hyoid bone.[5, 6]

According to a systematic review that investigated the performance of PMCT in fatal strangulation, autopsy demonstrated soft tissue hemorrhage in 33.8%, hyoid fracture in 21.7%, and thyroid cartilage fracture in 24.5% of the hanging cases.[3, 4] In fatal cases of manual strangulation, although only a few cases have been investigated, hemorrhage into subcutaneous tissue and neck muscle is the most common sign present in 80% of cases, followed by laryngeal and hyoid fractures (33.3%)[3, 7] However, Yen et al.[4] noted that lymph node hemorrhage may constitute frequent and specific evidence of fatal manual stran-

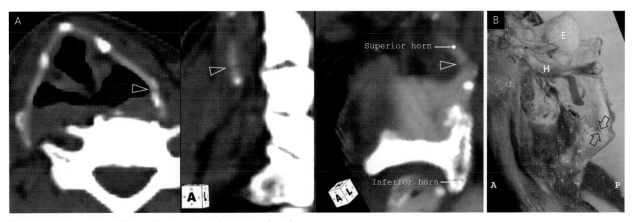

Figure 2. Thyroid cartilage fracture in a hanging death.
Axial (left), oblique coronal (middle), and oblique sagittal (right) images of postmortem CT demonstrate a fracture line and angulation of the left superior horn (arrowheads) of the thyroid cartilage (A), consistent with the findings during autopsy dissection (B). E: epiglottis, H: hyoid bone, A: anterior, P: posterior.

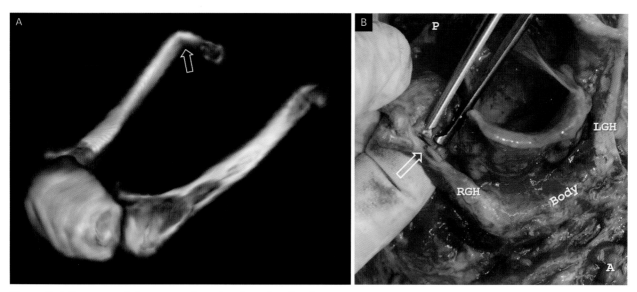

Figure 3. A Fracture of the greater horn in a hanging death.
Three-dimensional volume-rendered CT image (A) shows a focal fracture and angular deformity (arrow) of the right greater horn, which were confirmed during gross examination (arrow in B). In our experience, however, fractures of small bony structures are not always easily observed via CT unless fractured fragment displacement is evident.
LGH: left greater horn of bone, RGH: right greater horn of hyoid, A: anterior, P: posterior.

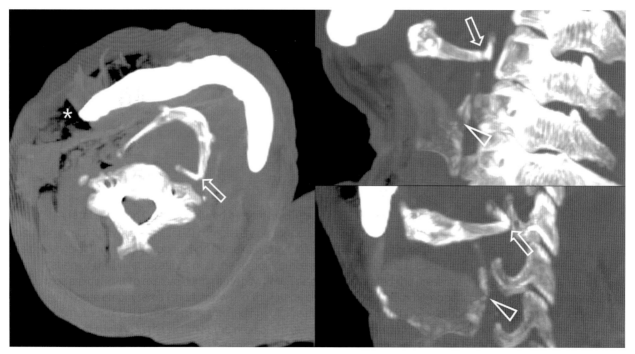

Figure 4. A 50-year-old male found decomposed.
Axial (left) and oblique sagittal (right) images of postmortem CT show fracture and deformity of the left greater horn (arrows) of hyoid bone and the ipsilateral superior horn of thyroid cartilage (arrowheads).

gulation. In ligature strangulation, soft tissue hemorrhage was found during autopsy in 41.7%, thyroid fracture in 25%, and hyoid fracture in 8.3% of cases.

PMCT has been used mainly for the investigation of fractures of the hyoid bone and thyroid cartilage in cases of strangulation fatality (Figs. 2-4). Compared with autopsy, PMCT has reportedly demonstrated almost equivalent or superior results with respect to the detection of thyroid cartilage fractures (25% vs. 25%) and hyoid bone fractures (24.2% vs. 21.0%) in cases of hanging, manual strangulation, and ligature strangulation.[3] However, PMCT is not suitable for detecting hemorrhages in the neck. PMCT reportedly missed many soft tissue hemorrhages, which were found with more than twofold greater frequency during autopsy (38.2%) than during PMCT (16.9%). In contrast, although few cases have been investigated, postmortem MR imaging is nearly equivalent to autopsy for the detection of soft tissue hemorrhage. [3, 4] PMCT is a reliable tool for the detection of gas accumulation in cases of fatal strangulation. Pneumomediastinum and soft tissue emphysema can be easily detected by PMCT, but they may not be readily noticed during conventional autopsy.[8] This soft tissue gas is presumed to originate from the rupture of highly pressurized alveoli by hanging; it is reportedly present in more than one-fourth of all hanging cases.[3] The detection of hemorrhage and gas accumulation within soft tissue are considered to be vital reactions in cases of strangulation: evidence of vitality in the victim prior to the event.

Traumatic spondylolisthesis of the axis (i.e., hangman's fracture) is a common hyperextension injury of the cervical spine caused by bilateral fractures of the pars interarticularis, which generally occur during motor vehicle accidents and falls from height.[9, 10] In contrast to its informal name, this pattern of fracture is rarely found in cases of hanging and only observed in approximately 10% of judicial hanging deaths[9, 11], which have adopted a standard or long drop (i.e., drop of > 1.2 m). In this type of hanging, the injury is caused by body weight/knot positioning, as well as the drop length. However, the actual incidence and circumstance of this type of fracture in cases of hanging have been debated for many decades.[10]

Hanging is a common method of suicide, as well as judicial punishment.[12] Suicide or nonjudicial hanging usually involves full suspension of the body using a raised support (e.g., a chair, ladder, or cart) with a rope around the neck. Partial suspension is also commonly used for this type of hanging. In these instances, the victim exhibits self-ligation around the neck and both feet, or may exhibit knees touching the ground in a partial weight-bearing position. Hangman's fracture can be observed in nonjudicial hanging involving a long drop (e.g., jump from a bridge with a rope around the neck).[10, 13] Although rare, hangman's fracture can be clearly identified by PMCT, including the bony fracture itself, hemorrhage into the soft tissue, and subarachnoid hemorrhage in the spinal canal and basal cistern. PMCT is useful for detecting fracture of the C2 vertebral body, particularly for cases without disc rupture and angulation or displacement of fractured fragments. Fractures without displacement generally can escape autopsy unless bleeding is evident in the surrounding tissue.[10, 14]

References

1   Sauvageau A, Boghossian E. Classification of asphyxia: the need for standardization. Journal of forensic sciences. 2010;55(5):1259-67. doi: 10.1111/j.1556-4029.2010.01459.x.

2   Sauvageau A. About strangulation and hanging: Language matters. Journal of emergencies, trauma, and shock. 2011;4(2):320. doi: 10.4103/0974-2700.82238.

3   Gascho D, Heimer J, Tappero C, Schaerli S. Relevant findings on postmortem CT and postmortem MRI in hanging, ligature strangulation and manual strangulation and their additional value compared to autopsy - a systematic review. Forensic science, medicine, and pathology. 2019;15(1):84-92. doi: 10.1007/s12024-018-0070-z.

4   Yen K, Thali MJ, Aghayev E, Jackowski C, Schweitzer W, Boesch C, et al. Strangulation signs: initial correlation of MRI, MSCT, and forensic neck findings. Journal of magnetic resonance imaging : JMRI. 2005;22(4):501-10. doi: 10.1002/jmri.20396.

5   Nikolic S, Micic J, Atanasijevic T, Djokic V, Djonic D. Analysis of neck injuries in hanging. The American journal of forensic medicine and pathology. 2003;24(2):179-82. doi: 10.1097/01.PAF.0681069550.31660.f5.

6   Green H, James RA, Gilbert JD, Byard RW. Fractures of the hyoid bone and laryngeal cartilages in suicidal hanging. Journal of clinical forensic medicine. 2000;7(3):123-6. doi: 10.1054/jcfm.2000.0419.

7   Decker LA, Hatch GM, Lathrop SL, Nolte KB. The Role of Postmortem Computed Tomography in the Evaluation of Strangulation Deaths. Journal of forensic sciences. 2018;63(5):1401-5. doi: 10.1111/ 1556-4029.13760.

8   Lee H, Lee S, Cha JG, Baek T, Yang KM. Postmortem Computed Tomography and Computed Tomography Angiography: Cardiothoracic Imaging Applications in Forensic Medicine. Journal of thoracic imaging. 2019;34(5):286-98. doi: 10.1097/rti.0000000000000398.

9   Murphy H, Schroeder GD, Shi WJ, Kepler CK, Kurd MF, Fleischman AN, et al. Management of Hangman's Fractures: A Systematic Review. Journal of orthopaedic trauma. 2017;31 Suppl 4:S90-s5. doi: 10.1097/bot.0000000000000952.

10   Hayashi T, Hartwig S, Tsokos M, Oesterhelweg L. Postmortem multislice computed tomography (pmMSCT) imaging of hangman's fracture. Forensic science, medicine, and pathology. 2014;10(1):3-8. doi: 10.1007/s12024-013-9430-x.

11   James R, Nasmyth-Jones R. The occurrence of cervical fractures in victims of judicial hanging. Forensic science international. 1992; 54(1):81-91. doi: 10.1016/0379-0738(92)90083-9.

12   Wallace SK, Cohen WA, Stern EJ, Reay DT. Judicial hanging: postmortem radiographic, CT, and MR imaging features with autopsy confirmation. Radiology. 1994;193(1):263-7. doi: 10.1148/radiology.193.1.8090904.

13   Amadasi A, Buschmann CT, Tsokos M. Complex fracture patterns in hanging associated with a fall from height. Forensic science, medicine, and pathology. 2020;16(2):359-61. doi: 10.1007/s12024-019-00210-6.

14   Gerlock AJ, Jr., Mirfakhraee M. Computed tomography and hangman's fractures. Southern medical journal. 1983;76(6):727-8. doi: 10.1097/00007611-198306000-00012.

Chapter 08

Drowning

Drowning is a form of fatal asphyxia caused by protracted submersion of the face in a liquid, usually water, and aspiration of the liquid into the airway. According to the World Health Organization, up to 372,000 individuals worldwide die annually because of drowning.[1] During the period 2015-2019, the Korean Statistical Information Service reported that the mean numbers of drowning-related accidental and suicidal deaths in Korea were both 570 per year.[2]

Drowning is a cause of death that is difficult to establish with traditional autopsy due to its nonspecific postmortem findings.[3, 4] When a corpse is found in water, there are several possible scenarios, thus raising the critical question of whether the individual entered the water while alive or after death.[5] Drowning is diagnosed on the basis of circumstantial evidence (e.g., public surveillance camera, police records, and/or eyewitness testimony) and some typical but nonspecific autopsy findings: frothy foam in the upper airway (mouth and nasal cavities) and enlarged lungs due to both pulmonary edema and

excessive expansion caused by the inhalation of air and water. Although the aspiration of either freshwater or saltwater can lead to pulmonary edema, several studies have illustrated the distinction between saltwater and freshwater drowning.[6] The hypertonicity of aspirated saltwater reportedly causes fluid to be drawn from circulation into the interstitium and alveoli, leading to hypovolemia, hypertonic serum, and pulmonary edema. In contrast, hypotonic freshwater rapidly passes through the alveolar membrane into the intravascular compartment, leading to volume overload and hemodilution. Therefore, it is difficult to understand why pulmonary edema occurs in cases of drowning or near-drowning in freshwater. A potential influencing factor is the abnormal surfactant property, particularly in freshwater drowning, which may cause increased alveolar permeability and instability.[7] In addition, transient circulatory volume overload and neurogenic cause is presumed to influence the development of pulmonary edema in cases of freshwater drowning.[8]

However, these findings may also be observed in individuals who have died of other causes (e.g., asphyxia, drug overdose, or carbon monoxide poisoning)[3-5], although the severities of the findings may be reduced. Thus far, the detection of diatoms in the blood circulation and organs has been suggested as more reliable evidence of death by drowning, provided if there is no gross decomposition or traumatic injuries of the body. However, it is technically difficult and negative results cannot exclude drowning. [9] From a forensic perspective, therefore, drowning is considered a diagnosis of exclusion (i.e., a diagnosis made after excluding other potential causes of death).[3]

In recent years, there have been many reports regarding the use of postmortem CT to obtain imaging data in cases of drowning.[3-5, 10-13] Postmortem CT (PMCT) is particularly useful to detect water inflow into the paranasal sinuses and mastoid air cells, which is difficult to identify via classic autopsy. [3] Previous studies.[5, 10, 11] have indicated that fluid in the paranasal sinuses is most often detected in the maxillary (98-100%) and sphenoidal sinuses (88-100%), followed by the ethmoidal (80-100%) and frontal (70-100%) sinuses. Furthermore, fluid density in the paranasal sinuses can be used to differentiate between saltwater and freshwater drowning. Specifically, sinus fluid has a greater mean density in saltwater drowning (47 HU) than in freshwater drowning (33 HU) [14], although further studies with additional cases are needed to confirm these findings. PMCT is also useful for quantifying pulmonary edema. Ground-glass opacity with interstitial thickening, ill-defined centrilobular nodules along the airway, and the combination of these two manifestations are the most frequent findings, present in 86% of all cases. Ground-glass opacities originate mostly from partial alveolar filling with fluid; reticular opacities reportedly represent a thickened interlobular septum caused by the accumulation of edematous fluid in interstitial spaces; and centrilobular nodules with patchy alveolar densities may imply the aspiration of both freshwater (**Figs. 1 and 2**) and saltwater (**Figs. 3-5**).[15-17]

PMCT can be used to evaluate emphysema aquosum, a waterlogged state of lung hyperinflation caused by a check valve-type blockage of the upper airways while inhaling a combination of air and water.[3, 4] Overinflation of the lungs can be indirectly quantified on PMCT. In one study, the mean level of the right hemidiaphragm in drowning victims reached 5.32 according to the anterior rib levels due to lung expansion, compared with 4.56 in the non-drowning strangulation group.[5] Furthermore, in a study regarding death by freshwater drowning, the hemodilution effect caused by the rapid absorption of hypotonic water into circulation was visible on CT images as a reduction in cardiac chamber density.[13]

Most prior studies suggested that these CT findings were indicative of drowning after comparison with findings from other causes of death (e.g., sudden cardiac death or fatal brain injury). However, one recent study[4], implied that these imaging findings are not specific to drowning, and suggested that any specific findings are indicative of "asphyxia", rather than "drowning" alone. There were no statistically significant findings specific to drowning alone, when compared with the findings from other types of asphyxiation (e.g., strangulation, compressive or positional asphyxia, choking, and smothering). However,

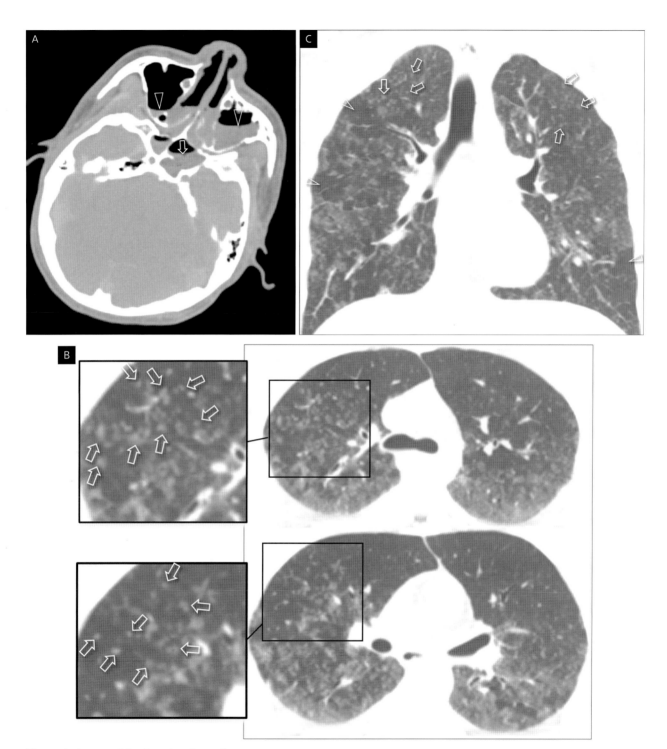

Figure 1. A case of freshwater drowning

Postmortem CT of a male victim found dead in a rainwater pumping station shows fluid collection in the sphenoid (arrow) and maxillary sinuses (arrowheads) in an axial (A) image of the head. Axial (B) and coronal (C) images with lung window setting show numerous ill-defined centrilobular nodules (arrows in magnified images of B) in both lungs, indicative of fluid collection in small bronchioles. Note the presence of multifocal subpleural low densities (arrowheads) suggestive of lobular air trappings (arrowheads in C).

another study investigated whether CT findings in cases of drowning can reliably distinguish between drowning and strangulation by hanging.[5] In that study, the significantly more frequent findings in cases of drowning (compared with hanging) included excessive fluid in the paranasal sinuses (up to 98%), upper airway and trachea (78-98%), pleural cavity (71%) and pericardial cavity (59%), as well as luminal distention in the gastrointestinal tract, particularly the esophagus (81%), stomach (71%), duodenum (34%), and jejunum (31%).

It is reasonable that the discovery of a body in water does not automatically implicate drowning as the cause of death. To determine that death occurred from drowning, evidence from various sources should be considered.[4] Accordingly, some CT findings may support the diagnosis of drowning, despite substantial overlap between the imaging features of drowning and other causes of death. For example, the presence of fluid in the paranasal sinuses has low positive predictive value; however, the absence of this finding may exclude drowning with a high level of certainty.[4, 12] As demonstrated in the above cases, PMCT allows the examination of anatomical areas that are not easily accessible in conventional autopsy and thus provides further information during the death investigation.[18]

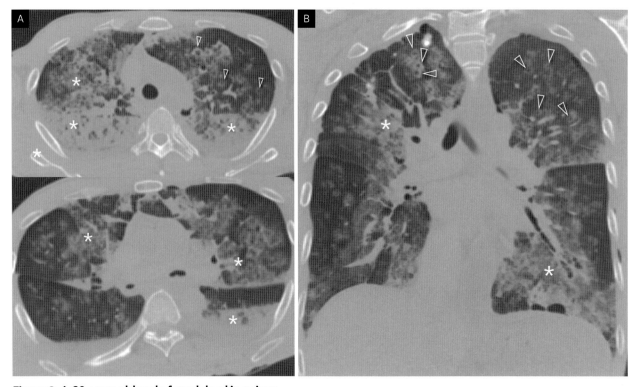

Figure 2. A 60-year-old male found dead in a river.
Axial (A) and coronal (B) postmortem CT images of the lungs demonstrate bronchial wall thickening (arrowheads) and a mixed pattern of ground-glass opacities (GGOs) and consolidation (*) with peribronchial distribution. Note the bilateral horizontal borders of mixed GGOs and consolidation, indicative of the postmortem sedimentation of aspirated water.

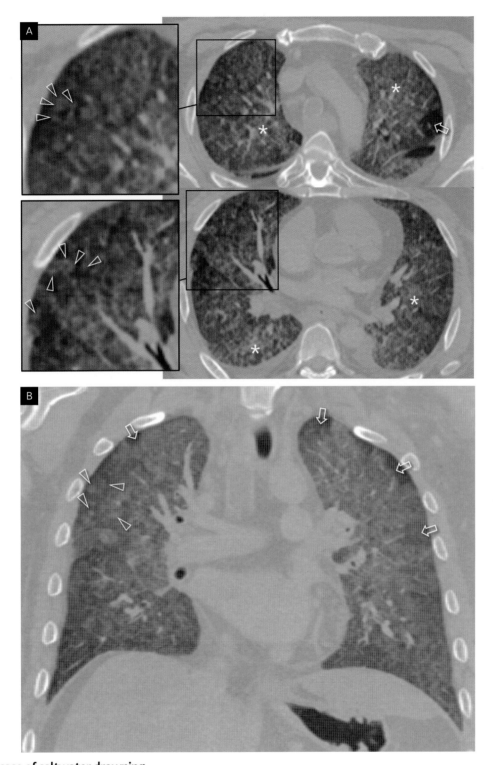

Figure 3. A case of saltwater drowning

Axial (A) and coronal (B) Postmortem CT images of the lungs show ill-defined centrilobular nodules (arrowheads in magnified images of A and B) and patchy ground-glass opacities (*), predominantly with subpleural and central distributions. Note the presence of multifocal subpleural low densities (arrows in B), indicative of air trapping due to bronchiolar occlusion.

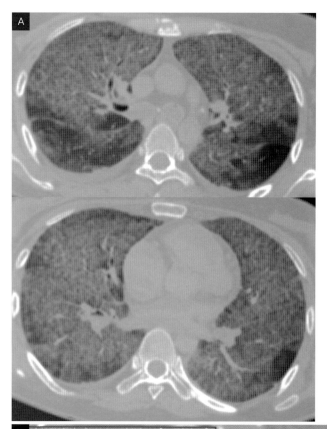

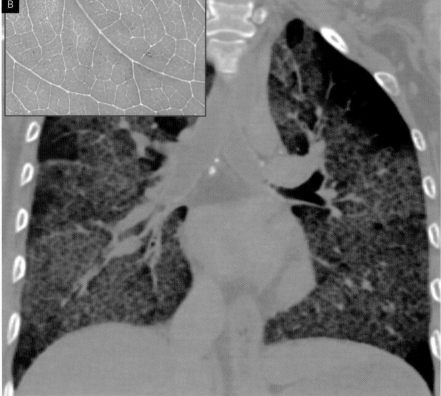

Figure 4. A dead body found floating in the sea.
Postmortem CT of a 43-year-old female shows reticular patterns of interstitial densities with intra- and interlobular septal thickenings on axial (A) and coronal (B) images of the lungs, indicative of pulmonary edema. Leaf venation (small box in B) shows a reticular pattern, similar to the thickened interstitial lung markings.

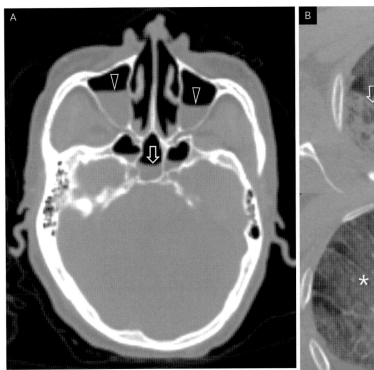

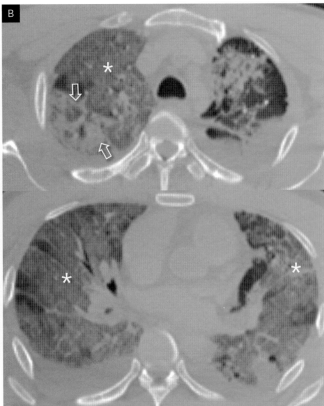

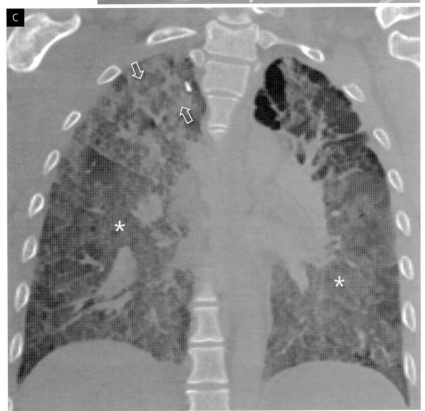

Figure 5. A saltwater drowning victim found dead in the sea.

Postmortem CT of a 45-year-old male found dead in the sea shows fluid collection in the sphenoid (arrow) and maxillary sinuses (arrowheads) in an axial (A) image of the head. Axial (upper and lower in B) and coronal (C) images of the lungs show a mixed pattern of patchy consolidations (arrows) and ground-glass opacities (*), suggestive of pulmonary edema and fluid aspiration.

References

1   World Health Organization. Global Report on Drowning: Preventing a Leading Killer. World Health Organization; 2014.

2   Korean Statistical Information Service. Cause of death statistics. (2015-2019).

3   Usui A, Kawasumi Y, Funayama M, Saito H. Postmortem lung features in drowning cases on computed tomography. Japanese journal of radiology. 2014;32(7):414-20. doi: 10.1007/s11604-014-0326-9.

4   Van Hoyweghen AJ, Jacobs W, Op de Beeck B, Parizel PM. Can post-mortem CT reliably distinguish between drowning and non-drowning asphyxiation? International journal of legal medicine. 2015;129(1):159-64. doi: 10.1007/s00414-014-1037-6.

5   Vander Plaetsen S, De Letter E, Piette M, Van Parys G, Casselman JW, Verstraete K. Post-mortem evaluation of drowning with whole body CT. Forensic science international. 2015;249:35-41. doi: 10.1016/j.forsciint.2015.01.008.

6   Battaglia JD, Lockhart CH. Drowning and near-drowning. Pediatric annals. 1977;6(4):270-5.

7   Layon AJ, Modell JH. Drowning: Update 2009. Anesthesiology. 2009;110(6):1390-401. doi: 10.1097/ALN.0b013e3181a4c3b8.

8   Rumbak MJ. The etiology of pulmonary edema in fresh water near-drowning. The American journal of emergency medicine. 1996; 14(2):176-9. doi: 10.1016/s0735-6757(96)90128-x.

9   Pollanen MS. The diagnostic value of the diatom test for drowning, II. Validity: analysis of diatoms in bone marrow and drowning medium. Journal of forensic sciences. 1997;42(2):286-90.

10 Levy AD, Harcke HT, Getz JM, Mallak CT, Caruso JL, Pearse L, et al. Virtual autopsy: two- and three-dimensional multidetector CT findings in drowning with autopsy comparison. Radiology. 2007; 243(3):862-8. doi: 10.1148/radiol.2433061009.

11 Christe A, Aghayev E, Jackowski C, Thali MJ, Vock P. Drowning-post-mortem imaging findings by computed tomography. European radiology. 2008;18(2):283-90. doi: 10.1007/s00330-007-0745-4.

12 Kawasumi Y, Kawabata T, Sugai Y, Usui A, Hosokai Y, Sato M, et al. Assessment of the relationship between drowning and fluid accumulation in the paranasal sinuses on post-mortem computed tomography. European journal of radiology. 2012;81(12):3953-5. doi: 10.1016/j.ejrad.2012.08.011.

13 Ambrosetti MC, Barbiani C, El-Dalati G, Pellini E, Raniero D, De Salvia A, et al. Virtual autopsy using multislice computed tomography in forensic medical diagnosis of drowning. La Radiologia medica. 2013;118(4):679-87. doi: 10.1007/s11547-012-0910-y.

14 Kawasumi Y, Usui A, Sato Y, Sato Y, Daigaku N, Hosokai Y, et al. Distinction between saltwater drowning and freshwater drowning by assessment of sinus fluid on post-mortem computed tomography. European radiology. 2016;26(4):1186-90. doi: 10.1007/s00330-015-3909-7.

15 Storto ML, Kee ST, Golden JA, Webb WR. Hydrostatic pulmonary edema: high-resolution CT findings. AJR American journal of roentgenology. 1995;165(4):817-20. doi: 10.2214/ajr.165.4.7676973.

16 Webb WR. Thin-section CT of the secondary pulmonary lobule: anatomy and the image--the 2004 Fleischner lecture. Radiology. 2006;239(2):322-38. doi: 10.1148/radiol.2392041968.

17 Gruden JF, Webb WR, Warnock M. Centrilobular opacities in the lung on high-resolution CT: diagnostic considerations and pathologic correlation. AJR American journal of roentgenology. 1994;162(3): 569-74. doi: 10.2214/ajr.162.3.8109498.

18 Lee H, Lee S, Cha JG, Baek T, Yang KM. Postmortem Computed Tomography and Computed Tomography Angiography: Cardiothoracic Imaging Applications in Forensic Medicine. Journal of thoracic imaging. 2019;34(5):286-98. doi: 10.1097/rti.0000000000000398.

Nontraumatic death

Chapter 09

Deaths by natural causes

What is "normal" and what is a "disease," after all?
The answer turns out to be very much dependent on historical context.
– HR Moody. Generations. 2001/2002;35;33–37

Natural death refers to the final result of a naturally occurring disease process or internal dysfunction of the body which results in death at a certain point.[1, 2] By definition, natural death does not occur from violence, an intended act (e.g., suicide), or an accident. Common causes of natural death include ischemic heart disease, cerebrovascular accident (stroke), respiratory disease, and infection.[3] However, in general, death investigations of those cases are not subject to forensic autopsy dissections because their deaths are "natural" and already anticipated, particularly in older people or patients with known chronic diseases.[4, 5] Therefore, investigations of natural deaths are usually performed in sudden or unexpected cases. Sudden death refers to an unexpected death that occurs "naturally" within 24 h after symptoms appear (International Classification of Diseases (ICD-10), World Health Organization, Geneva;2005). Moreover, sudden cardiac death (SCD) is clinically defined as death due to the loss of cardiac function, which occurs < 1 h after symptom onset.

[6-8] Sudden death is most commonly associated with cardiovascular disease attributed to atherosclerotic coronary artery disease, followed by other types of cardiovascular disease (e.g., hypertrophic cardiomyopathy), aortic disease (e.g., aneurysmal rupture and dissection)[7-11], cerebrovascular disease, pulmonary embolism, and asthma.[4, 12]

For the investigation of suspected natural death, the major roles of postmortem CT (PMCT) are to identify lethal pathologies that may lead to death, to screen for other potential causes of death that are "unnatural" (e.g., traumatic injuries) (Fig. 1), and to guide pathologists in the confirmation of such pathologies during subsequent autopsy dissection.

Thus far, PMCT has been generally recognized as a useful diagnostic supplement for forensic practice and incorporated as a routine procedure in many medicolegal institutions worldwide. Currently, it is intended to provide minimally-invasive, observer-independent, and reproducible death investigations that complement conventional autopsy. In addition,

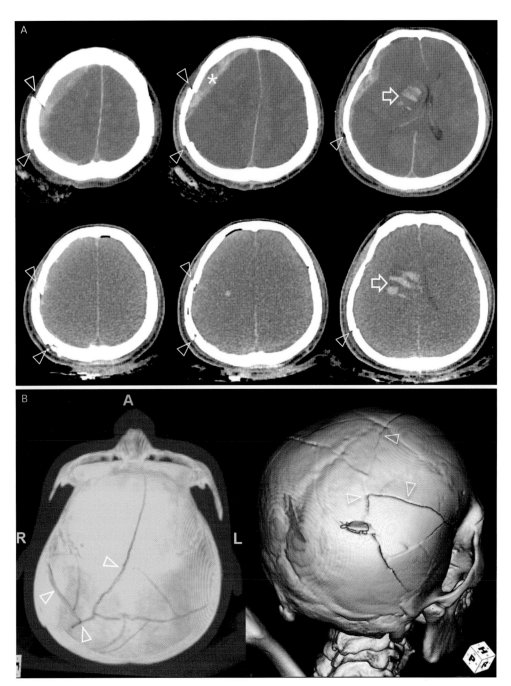

Figure 1. A case of intracerebral hemorrhage (ICH) followed by secondary traumatic subdural hematoma (SDH).
(A) Axial images of antemortem CT (upper row) shows acute hemorrhage (arrow) in the right basal ganglia and ipsilateral subdural hematoma (*) with adjacent skull fractures (arrowheads), suggestive of acute hypertensive ICH and secondary traumatic SDH. On postmortem CT (lower row) taken 3 days later, hemorrhage remains evident in the right basal ganglia, although the subdural hematoma was externally drained out through the fracture site (arrowheads). Note the presence of postmortem changes in the brain parenchyma, indicating the loss of gray-white matter differentiation and swelling of the brain. See Chapter 12 for the details of postmortem changes. (B) Minimum intensity projection (left) and three-dimensional volume-rendered (right) images of the calvarium show spiderweb fractures (arrowheads) of the vertex and high occiput (arrow), characteristic of a fall-related injury to the skull.

postmortem angiography (i.e., PMCT angiography {PMCTA}) has been introduced to address difficult forensic questions regarding the presence of critical vascular pathologies through explorations of the vascular system, to identify vascular ruptures or occlusions that are difficult or impossible to observe during autopsy dissection.[13-15] In this chapter, the current roles of PMCT and PMCTA are introduced in the evaluation of natural death by describing various diseases at different positions in the body.

9.1. Coronary Artery and Heart

Currently, cardiovascular diseases remain the most common causes of natural death in many developed countries. While SCD is generally attributable to myocardial ischemia consequent to coronary artherosclerosis and its complications[7], hypertrophic cardiomyopathy is a more frequent cause of SCD in athletes <35 years of age.[9, 16] The most common autopsy findings, identified in 80% of SCD victims, are atherosclerotic plaques and associated luminal stenosis (more than 75% of cross-sectional area in one or more coronary arteries), which is generally regarded as hemodynamically significant.[8-11, 17]

Coronary obstruction by thrombi and ruptured plaques are found in 20-70% of SCD victims.[8] However, the proposed mechanism of death in SCD victims is fatal arrhythmia (e.g., ventricular fibrillation/tachyarrhythmia, bradyarrhythmia, or asystole) [9], which is caused by acute ischemic myocardial changes that may include myocardial infarction or not.[8, 9, 18] Therefore, it is essential to understand

that diagnosis of SCD can be determined in the presence of diffuse and non-occlusive coronary artery disease, regardless of myocardial infarction, after strict exclusion of non-cardiac causes of death.[8, 9, 19] If SCD is suspected, visualization of the coronary artery and its luminal patency is critical considerations.[20] Nonenhanced CT can detect and quantify the coronary calcium, which can be used as an indicator of total plaque burden. This characteristic is used to estimate cardiovascular risk and predict future cardiac events in clinical setting.[21, 22] However, intravascular contrast injection is needed to identify noncalcified plaque or thromboembolic occlusion, and to assess the degree of luminal stenosis.[10, 23] Although the coronary calcium burden is reportedly related to total atherosclerotic burden, it is not proportional to the degree of luminal stenosis. In addition, the absence of coronary artery calcium on CT does not imply the absence of noncalcified plaques, thrombotic coronary occlusion by plaque rupture, or coronary artery embolism (Fig. 2).[21, 22]

In this regard, PMCT has showed promising results following intravascular contrast injection. In particular, PMCTA allows the direct visualization of coronary arteries and heart structures, demonstrating coronary plaques or thrombi, luminal stenosis or obstruction (Figs. 3-5), and myocardial rupture (Fig. 6), including in highly decomposed bodies (Fig. 7).

An additional advantage of PMCTA is its ability to detect both long and short lengths of substantial stenosis that could be missed by large interval sections of gross specimens[7], with minimal likelihood of displacing antemortem thrombi using injection pressure lower than perfusion pressure in living pa-

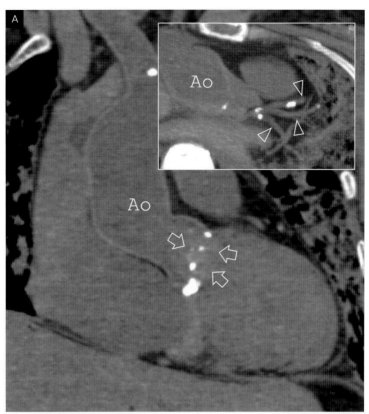

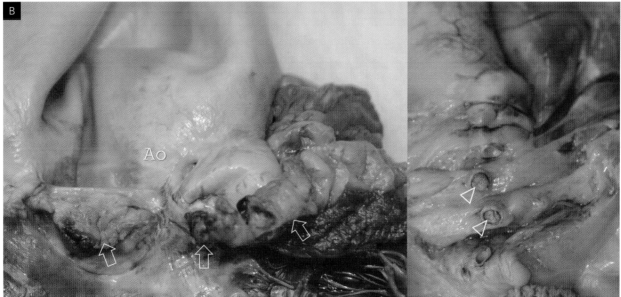

Figure 2. A 69-year-old female with infective endocarditis complicated by fatal left coronary artery embolization.
(A) Oblique coronal image of postmortem CT shows aortic valvular thickening and calcifications, but does not depict luminal abnormalities of the coronary arteries (arrowheads) due to the lack of contrast enhancement of vascular lumen (axial image in small box). (B) Photography of pathological specimen reveals aortic vegetations (arrows) and embolic occlusion (arrowheads) of the left anterior descending coronary artery. Ao: aorta.

Image B adapted from sudden cardiac death caused by a septic coronary artery embolism (accepted) by Kim et al., with permission of Korean J Leg Med.

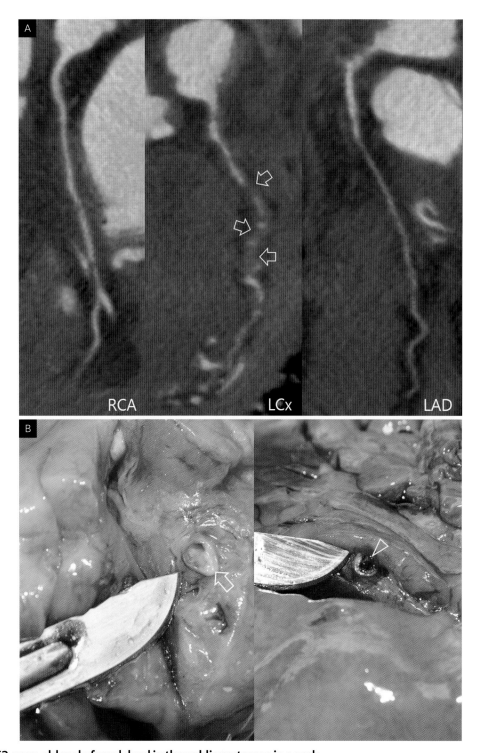

Figure 3. A 53-year-old male found dead in the public restroom in a park.

(A) Curved multiplanar reconstruction images of postmortem CT angiography show irregular stenosis (arrows) of the LCx caused by extensive thrombus. (B) Cross-sectional views of the LCx shows atherosclerotic plaque (arrow in left) and extensive thrombus (arrowhead in right) with > 75% stenosis.

LCx: left circumflex coronary artery.

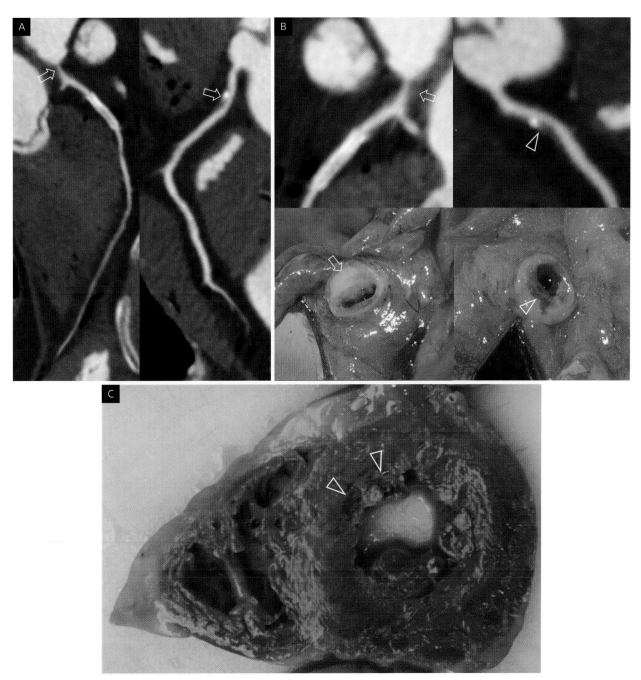

Figure 4. A 63-year-old male found dead 5 days after coronary stent placement in the left anterior descending artery (LAD).
(A) Curved multiplanar images of postmortem CT angiography show a patent stent in the proximal LAD, but severe (90%) stenosis of the left main coronary artery (LM, arrow in left) and moderate (50%) stenosis of the proximal segment of the right coronary artery (RCA, arrow in right). (B) Magnified CT images focusing on the LM artery (upper left) and proximal RCA (upper right) show stenosis caused by noncalcified plaque (arrows) and mixed plaque (arrowhead), respectively, which were subsequently identified as lipid plaque (arrow in lower left) and fibrous plaque (arrowhead in lower right), respectively, during autopsy dissection. (C) Specimen photography of the heart shows a subacute stage endocardial infarction (arrowheads) in the anterior wall of the left ventricle.

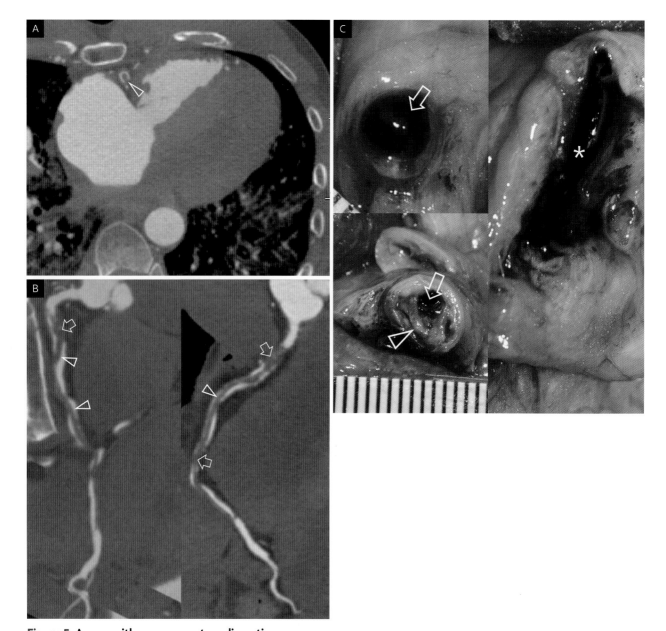

Figure 5. A case with coronary artery dissection.

(A) Axial image of postmortem CT angiography shows a dissection flap in the middle segment of the RCA. (B) Curvilinear reformation images of postmortem CT angiography show dissection of the RCA with dissection flaps (arrows) extending from the proximal segment to the middle segment. Note the presence of multifocal thrombosis (arrowheads) in the false lumen of the RCA. (C) Autopsy photograph of the RCA shows coronary artery dissection and thrombosis in the false lumen (arrows). Note the collapse of the true lumen (arrowhead) and thrombus (*) removed from the false lumen. RCA: right coronary artery

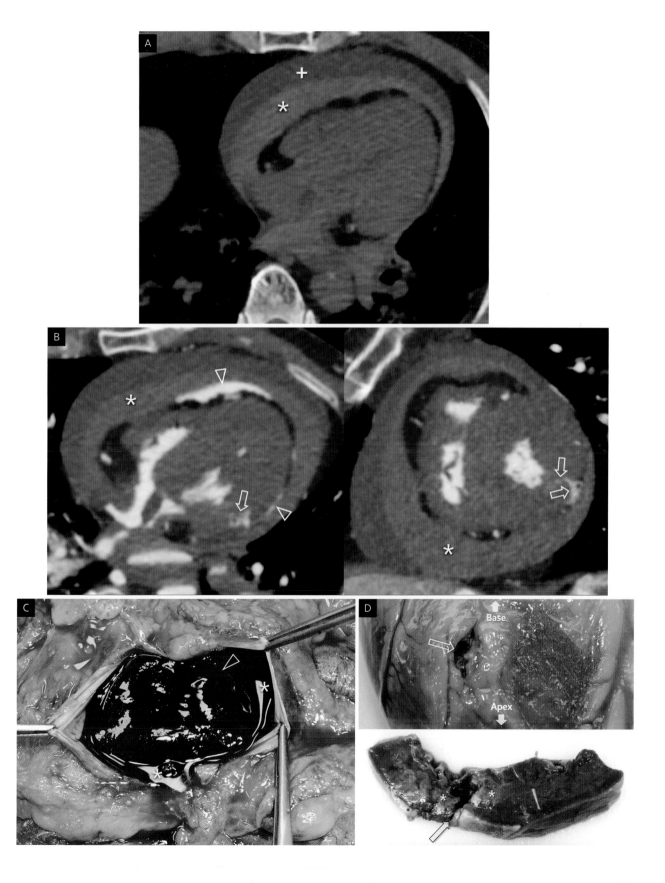

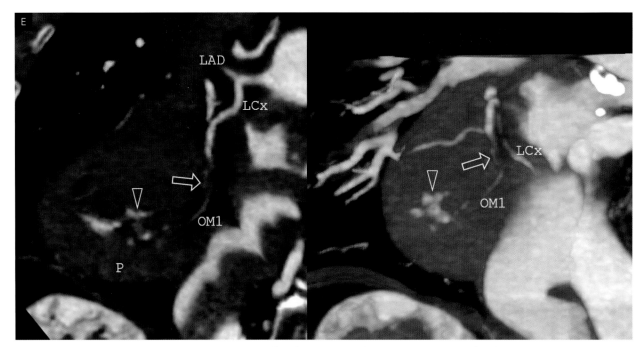

Figure 6. Myocardial rupture in a 64-year-old male who was found dead and presumed to have collapsed while washing his car.

(A) Axial image of PMCT shows double concentric bands of hemopericardium, with a hypodense outer ring (+) and hyperdense inner ring (*) on the epicardial surface. This so-called hyperdense "armored heart" sign is generated by selective coagulation of blood on a pulsating epicardial surface. Compare with Figure 1 in Chapter 11. (B) Four-chamber (left) and short-axis (right) PMCTA images of the LV reveal a myocardial defect (arrow) and contrast agent leakage (arrowhead) into the pericardial cavity from the LV cavity, indicating myocardial rupture as the cause of intrapericardial hemorrhage, in combination with the inner hyperdense concentric layer (*) of hemopericardium. (C) After pericardium opening, autopsy photography demonstrated coagulated blood (arrowhead) surrounded by non-coagulated hemorrhage (*), which was responsible for the double-band appearance on PMCT and PMCTA. (D) Photographs of the pathology specimen show focal myocardial rupture (arrows) in the inferolateral wall of the LV (upper image) and a sectional cut of the injured myocardium (lower image). Note the presence of an infarcted area (*) around the myocardial rupture.
(E) Curved multiplanar reformatted image (left) and maximum intensity projection image (right) of PMCTA depict the site of myocardial rupture (arrowhead) and thrombotic occlusion of the obtuse marginal branch (arrow) of the LCx supplying the corresponding left ventricular myocardium. PMCT: postmortem CT, PMCTA: postmortem CT angiography, LV: left ventricle, LAD: left anterior descending artery, LCx: left circumflex artery, OM1: 1st obtuse marginal branch

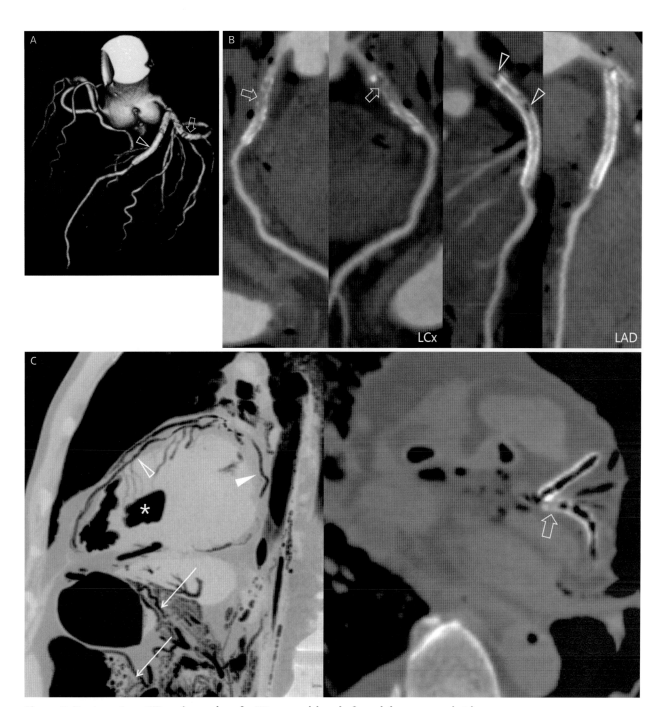

Figure 7. Postmortem CT angiography of a 53-year-old male found decomposed at home.
(A) 3D VR image shows a stent in LAD (arrowhead) and LCx (arrow), respectively. (B) Curved MPR images depict thrombotic occlusion of a stent (arrows) in the proximal LCx, but show a patent stent in the proximal LAD. Note the presence of air densities (arrowheads) in the lumen of the LAD stent, presumably due to decomposition. (C) MinIP image in oblique sagittal plane (left) reconstructed from nonenhanced CT shows extensive intravascular air collection by decomposition in the LAD (arrowhead), LCx (white arrowhead), and mesenteric vessels (long arrow), as well as the left ventricle (*). 3D VR: Three-dimensional volume-rendered, LAD: left anterior descending coronary artery, LCx: left circumflex coronary artery, MPR: multiplanar reformation, MinIP: minimal intensity projection.

tients.[10, 20] In contrast, using sufficient pressure for the expansion of a collapsed lumen, PMCTA has also been described as a better method to demonstrate the luminal patency of calcified coronary arteries, which would have otherwise been considered obstructed during autopsy.[7]

Thus far, primarily due to inherently low soft tissue resolution of CT, it has been difficult to describe the pathological nature of lesions that cause luminal stenosis. Therefore, histological examinations should determine the presence of hemorrhage and erosion, as well as the rupture of plaque with adjacent thrombus formation. In cases where PMCTA shows luminal stenosis of a coronary artery, It can be used for precise lesion localization, guiding the pathologist in histology sampling and facilitating the autopsy workflow. Furthermore, CT angiography is a morphological imaging method and does not reveal the functional importance of luminal narrowing identified in clinical practice.[7, 10] Similarly, vascular stenosis found on PMCTA alone is insufficient to determine fully the cause of death. For instance, the presence of tight stenosis on PMCTA does not reliably predict the presence of accompanying myocardial ischemia in the postmortem setting, as is not predicted by autopsy.[19] In real-world practice, however, the identification of cross-sectional stenosis more than 75% during autopsy and on PMCTA is regarded as a critical lesion with hemodynamic significance that may lead to acute ischemia and SCD, following careful exclusion of other potentially fatal pathologies.[8, 10] Regarding the diagnosis of ischemic changes in the heart, histological examination remains the reference standard for investigating

myocardial ischemia, which shows a time-dependent pattern.[10] Several studies have shown that PMCTA may delineate the potential area of myocardial infarction by showing "pathological" enhancement that is indirectly suggestive of ischemic necrosis; this sign is reportedly correlated with areas of subacute or old infarction on histological examination.[7, 10, 20] The underlying mechanism of myocardial enhancement and its importance are not well understood yet.[10, 19] Myocardial rupture occurs after infarction, trauma, or endocarditis, and sometimes even after cardiopulmonary resuscitation. Notably, myocardial rupture develops in approximately 1-3% of cases with myocardial infarction. Although rare, rupture is the most serious complication of myocardial ischemia, and constitutes the second leading cause of in-hospital death in myocardial infarction, occurring characteristically among individuals aged >55-60 years and at 1-7 days after ST elevation infarction.[24, 25]

PMCT can suggest myocardial rupture based on imaging findings that indicate intrapericardial hemorrhage. In this case, hemopericardium is characterized by dual concentric bands of outer hypodense and inner hyperdense rings generated from motion-induced selective coagulation on epicardial surfaces (i.e., "hyperdense armored heart sign"). This finding can be used as strong forensic evidence of heartbeat during bleeding into the pericardial cavity.[15, 26, 27] However, PMCTA allows direct localization of the rupture site through the injection of intravascular contrast agent. In Figure 6, PMCTA depicts myocardial rupture and stenosis of the coronary artery supplying the corresponding myocardium, which raises strong suspicion of ischemic myocardial injury as a cause of rupture. In this manner, PMCT and PMCTA can provide key information in a few relevant images in selected cases, allowing "at a glance" understanding of disease process that led to death.

9.2. Aorta

Aortic diseases that may lead to death include aortic aneurysm and dissection. Aortic dissection refers to a longitudinal separation of aortic media caused by a tear in the intimal layer, thus allowing blood to enter the medial layer and create false lumen.[28, 29] The dissection can spread from the initial entry tear proximally into the aortic valve and coro-

nary arteries, or distally into the thoracoabdominal aorta and its branches. Death occurs as a complication of impaired perfusion from the aortic branch to the heart or other vital organs, or due to blood loss from aortic rupture. Therefore, in cases involving the ascending aorta, the causes of death are coronary artery obstruction, aortic valvular insufficiency, or pericardial tamponade. In contrast, elevated blood pressure in the false lumen leads to dynamic compression or static occlusion of the branch vessels, resulting in end-organ ischemia and infarction.[28-30] Aortic aneurysm is defined as aortic dilatation to >50% more than the expected normal diameter (approximately 5.0 cm for ascending aorta, 4.0 cm for descending aorta, 3.75 cm at the level of the

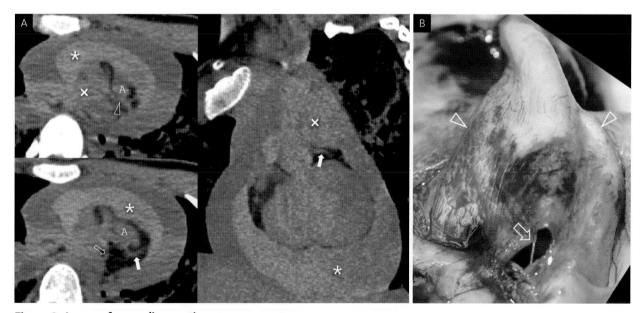

Figure 8. A case of ascending aortic aneurysm rupture.
(A) Axial (left) and oblique coronal (right) images of postmortem CT show hemopericardium with an inner hyperdense ring (*), indicative of intrapericardial hemorrhage before death and cardiac tamponade as the cause of death. Note the presence of hyperdense hemorrhage inside (x) and surrounding the mediastinum, suggesting a mediastinal source of hemorrhagic blood. Also note intact left main artery (arrowhead) and proximal segments of LAD (white-filled arrow) and LCx (arrow) embedded in epicardial fat. (B) Specimen photograph shows rupture (arrow) of the dilated ascending aorta (arrowheads) that caused hemopericardium in this case with suspected Marfan syndrome.

diaphragm, and 3.0 cm for abdominal aorta).[31-34] Although aortic aneurysms expand gradually and rarely cause specific symptoms, they result in aortic wall weakness and rupture, which can be life-threatening, mainly due to active and massive internal hemorrhage.

Without contrast enhancement, PMCT may demonstrate aortic contour deformity or high-density thrombus in the false lumen at acute stage of dissection. However, hemopericardium is the most common life-threatening complication of aortic dissection found on PMCT[4], and is identified by a "hyperdense armored heart" sign with a dense inner ring (Figs. 8 and 9).[27]

In most cases, however, PMCTA is required for pre-autopsy diagnosis of aortic dissection to identify intimal tearing and dissection flaps between the true and false lumens.

In cases with ruptured aortic aneurysm, noncontrast-enhanced PMCT may show the extravasation of blood into adjacent body cavities, as well as the ruptured aneurysm itself, but precise rupture localization is not possible without contrast enhancement. In cases where aneurysmal rupture is suspected, PMCTA shows the entire aorta (from ascending aorta to lower abdominal bifurcation), enabling the diagnostic classification of dissection and aneurysm, as well as the depiction of fatal complications.[15] For example, PMCTA evaluates the location of the entry tear, extension of the dissection flap, and presence of branch vessel occlusion in cases with aortic dissection. In cases with aortic aneurysm, PMCTA also provides further information regarding the size and location of lesions, as well as the presence of complications such as aortic rupture (Fig. 10), branch vessel occlusion, and end-organ ischemia.[13, 15]

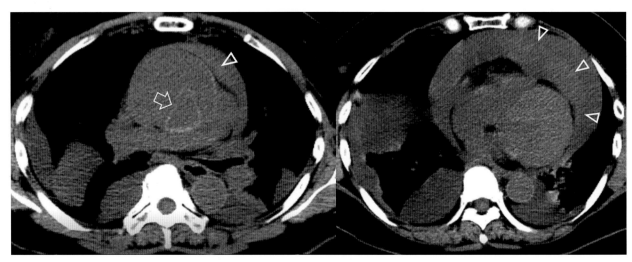

Figure 9. Antemortem CT of a case with ascending aortic aneurysm and Stanford class A aortic dissection.
Nonenhanced CT shows dissection flap (arrow) of the dilated ascending aorta and depicts hemopericardium with inner high-density crescent surrounding the heart (arrowheads), indicative of cardiac tamponade. Despite motion-induced artifacts from the heartbeat, CT successfully demonstrated the "hyperdense armored heart" sign in this case.

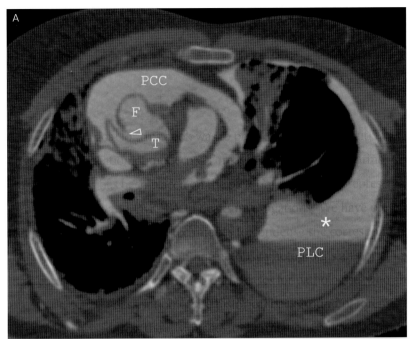

Figure 10. Postmortem CT angiography of a 66-year-old male with Stanford A class dissection. He was found dead at his bathroom.

Axial (A) and oblique coronal images (B) show a dissection flap between true (T) and false (F) lumens of ascending aorta and aortic arch, and depict the site of rupture (arrowhead) and contrast leakage into pericardial and pleural cavities, indicative of hemopericardium and hemothorax, respectively. In this case, a lipid-based contrast mixture lighter than blood was injected, which accumulated in the non-dependent position of the left pleural cavity (*in panel a).
PCC: pericardial cavity, PLC: pleural cavity, RA: right atrium, RV: right ventricle, LV: left ventricle, LA: left atrium.

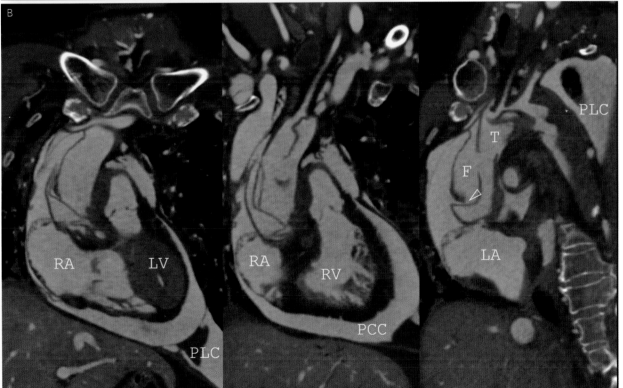

9.3. Cerebrovascular disease

Cerebrovascular accident (i.e., stroke or brain attack) is the second leading cause of death worldwide.[35] When blood flow to the brain is stopped by arterial occlusion or rupture, sudden brain cell death occurs due to oxygen deprivation.[36]

Stroke is composed of hemorrhagic and ischemic subtypes, which affect 10-20% and 80-90% of stroke cases, respectively.[37-39] Hemorrhagic stroke occurs when weakened vessels or aneurysms rupture either in the brain parenchyma (causing intracerebral hemorrhage, ICH) or into the subarachnoid space (causing subarachnoid hemorrhage, SAH).[37, 38] ICH is present in two-thirds of all hemorrhagic strokes and contributes to a higher mortality rate.[38, 40] Intracranial bleeding into or around the brain parenchyma produces tissue swelling and increases intracranial pressure, leading to brain damage and possible death.

In contrast, ischemic stroke is associated with either embolic or thrombotic obstruction of an intracranial cerebral artery. Notably, arterial occlusion in ischemic stroke is more frequently embolic (e.g., cardioembolic or arteroembolic). In cardioembolic stroke, arterial occlusion arises from the embolization of intracardiac thrombi associated with conditions such as atrial fibrillation or valvular disease. Arteroembolic strokes result from atherosclerotic disease in larger proximal arteries. In those cases, thrombus formation associated with plaque rupture in cervical carotid and vertebral arteries commonly leads to the distal embolization of thrombi, rather than on-site occlusion of diseased vessels. Thrombotic occlusion is a less common cause of ischemic stroke; it involves the on-site occlusion of intracranial arteries associated with atherosclerotic plaque rupture and subsequent thrombus formation.[39]

Although hemorrhagic stroke is less common, it causes up to 40% of all stroke-related deaths[40-43] and has a higher mortality rate, compared with ischemic stroke. Patients with hemorrhagic stroke survive for 1 year in 33% of ICH cases and 52% of SAH cases, respectively. In contrast, 77% of patients with ischemic stroke survive for 1 year.

The brain is highly susceptible to early postmortem changes such as autolysis and liquefaction, which begin immediately after death. Notably, these changes may conceal underlying pathologies or can be misidentified as true abnormalities on CT images. Therefore, it is vital to understand these "normal" postmortem processes in relation to their types, distributions, and times of onset. "Normal" postmortem changes in the brain include loss of gray-white matter differentiation and brain swelling with the effacement of ventricles and cisterns, beginning immediately after death.[13, 44, 45] However, these findings mostly depend on individual characteristics such as the victim's age and antemortem condition, length of agonal period, or environmental conditions.[45] As described earlier in this chapter, acute hemorrhage exhibits higher density, compared with brain parenchyma, on noncontrast CT images taken before or after death (**Figs. 11-14**) because of the high protein concentration (mainly globin molecules) in clotted blood. The high hemorrhage density, compared with the brain parenchyma density, allows CT to detect various degrees of hemorrhage in deeper and smaller structures that could be missed by large interval sec-

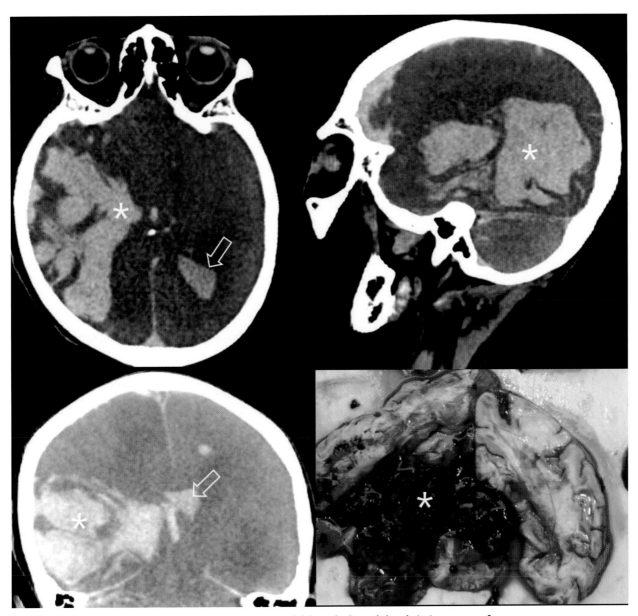

Figure 11. Intracerebral hemorrhage in an 83-year-old female found dead sitting on a sofa.
Axial (upper left), sagittal (upper right), and coronal (lower left) images of postmortem CT show high-density hemorrhage in the right basal ganglia and temporoparietal lobe (*), and in the left lateral ventricle (arrows). Autopsy photograph (lower right) demonstrates massive intracerebral hemorrhage in the right basal ganglia (*) and both lateral ventricles (arrow).

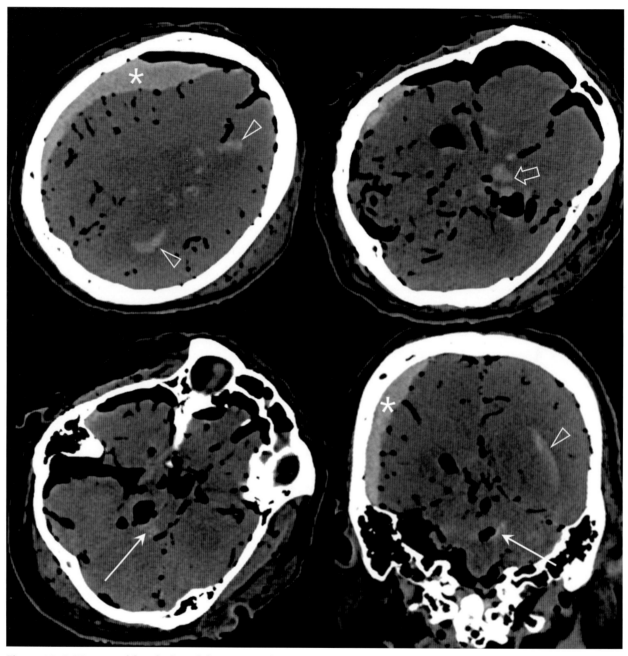

Figure 12. A 59-year-old male found decomposed.
Axial and coronal (lower right) images of postmortem CT demonstrate multifocal high-density hemorrhages in the right subdural space (*), left basal ganglia (arrow), and left lateral ventricle (arrowheads) in a moderately decomposed case. CT images also depict localized hemorrhage in the brainstem (long arrows). In this case, CT helps to infer a series of events in chronological order: focal hypertensive intracranial hemorrhage (arrow) of the left basal ganglia led to traumatic subdural hematoma (arrowhead) in the contralateral left hemisphere, which caused Duret hemorrhage in the brainstem due to elevated supratentorial pressure.

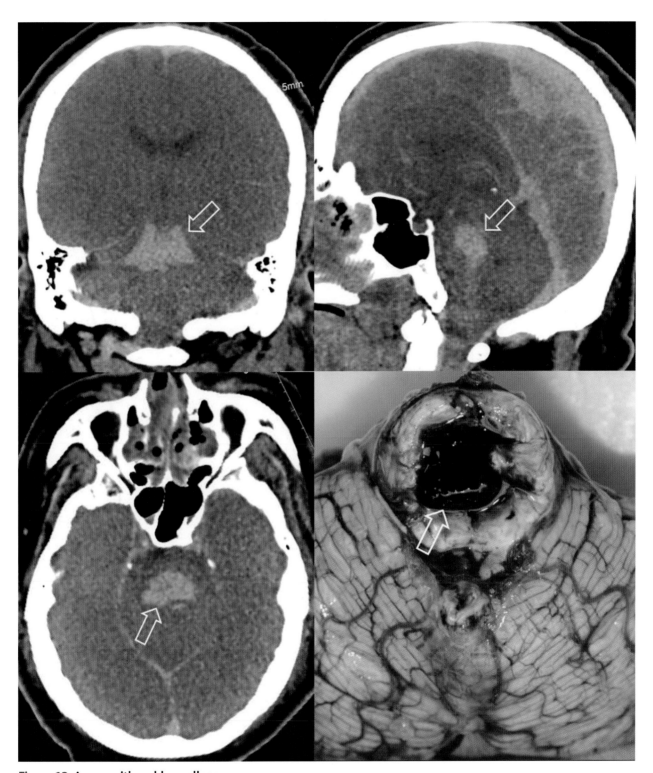

Figure 13. A case with sudden collapse.
Postmortem CT images show a high-density hemorrhage in the pons (arrow) in coronal (upper left), sagittal (upper right), and axial (lower left) images. Autopsy photograph of the brainstem demonstrates hemorrhage (arrow) in the pons.

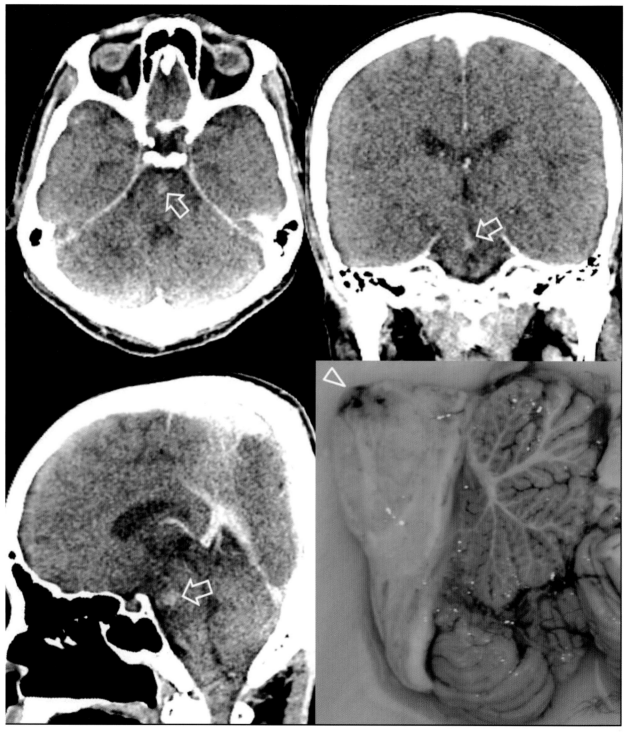

Figure 14. A case with pontine hemorrhage.
Postmortem CT images depict a small area of high density in the upper end of the pons in axial (upper left), coronal (upper right), and sagittal (lower left) images. Autopsy photograph shows minimal localized bleeding (arrow) in the pons, which corresponds to the bleeding area identified on CT. This small hemorrhage may be missed during sectioning of the specimen (arrowhead).

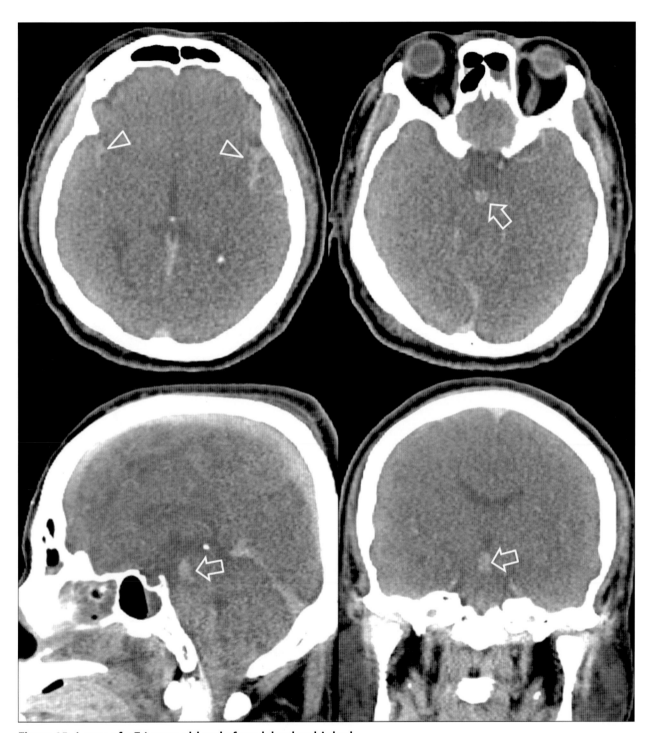

Figure 15. A case of a 54-year-old male found dead on his bed.

A small hemorrhage (arrow) of mid brain was found on axial (upper right), sagittal (lower left), and coronal (lower right) CT images. Note subarachnoid hemorrhage in the areas of both sylvian fissures (arrow heads in upper left), which might be originated from rupture of mid brain hemorrhage into subarachnoid space. As in this case, one advantage of PMCT would be its ability to detect even small but fatal hemorrhage particularly in the deep-seated structure vital for sustaining life.

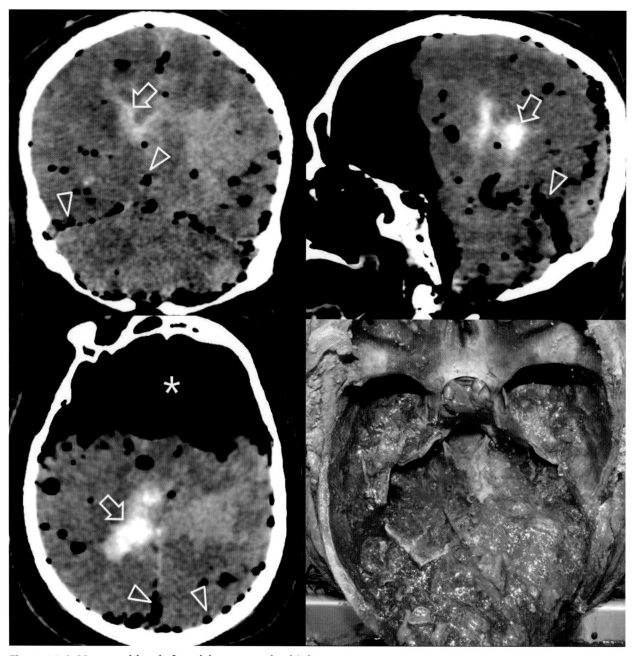

Figure 16. A 68-year-old male found decomposed at his home.

Postmortem CT demonstrates intracerebral hemorrhage (arrows) in coronal (upper left), sagittal (upper right), and axial (lower left) images. Note the presence of moderate to advanced decomposition of the brain with liquefaction and posterior settling, as well as putrefactive gas (* and arrowheads) in the cranial cavity. Autopsy photograph depicts partial liquefaction and softening of the brain with reddish discoloration, which interferes with the identification and localization of intracerebral hemorrhage during autopsy.

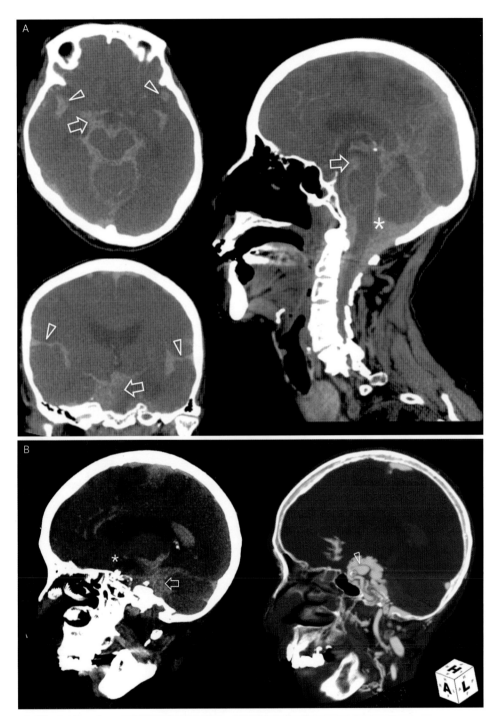

Figure 17. Postmortem CT and CT angiography of a case of cerebral aneurysm.

(A) Axial (left upper), coronal (left lower), and sagittal (right) images of postmortem CT shows subarachnoid hemorrhage at basal cistern (arrow), sylvian fissures (arrowheads), and posterior fossa (*). (B) Maximum intensity images in an oblique sagittal plane without (left) and with (right) intravascular contrast injection. Nonenhanced CT image shows acute stage of hematoma in basal cistern (arrow) but no aneurysm itself (*). Contrast enhanced image shows a contrast-filled aneurysmal sac (arrowhead) originated from the proximal position of the left middle cerebral artery, respectively. Note contrast leakage into the subarachnoid space, suggesting rupture of the aneurysmal sac.

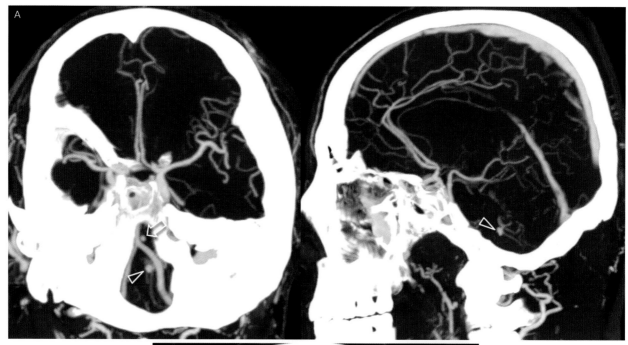

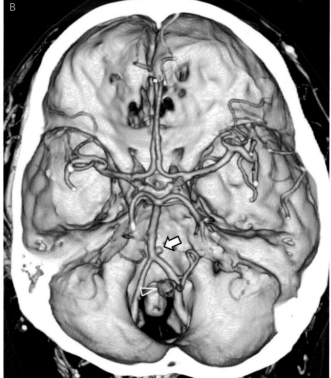

Figure 18. A case of incidental detection of an aneurysm of posterior circulation.
(A) Axial (left) and sagittal (right) maximal intensity projection images. (B) Three-dimensional volume-rendered image of the skull base. Postmortem CT angiography was performed on a 48-year-old male victim of a fatal stab wound and showed a tiny saccular aneurysm (arrows) of the basilar artery, immediately superior to the confluence of vertebral arteries, and an aneurysm (arrowheads) of posterior inferior cerebellar artery.

tions of gross specimens (**Fig. 15**).

In clinical CT imaging, hemorrhage density can be used to estimate the age of hemorrhagic blood; this density increases immediately after a bleeding event and reaches its maximum within a few hours due to clot formation and retraction. If the patient survives this acute period, the hemorrhage becomes isodense to surrounding brain parenchyma and difficult to detect over a few days to a few weeks. Eventually, its density gradually decreases to a level similar to that of water over a period of months.[46, 47] In contrast, the evolution of hemorrhage stops at the time of death because physiological breakdown of globin molecule ceases. This finding suggests that PMCT can be useful to identify intracranial hemorrhage, estimate the antemortem age of hemorrhagic blood at the time of death and, in severe cases, identify hemorrhage as a cause of death regardless of advanced decomposition (**Fig. 16**).[47]

PMCTA allows better gray-white matter differentiation in the brain. It has a great advantage in terms of noninvasive in situ representation of the intracranial vasculature, including posterior circulation. Injection of contrast material expands the vascular lumens that become collapsed after death, thereby allowing detection of atherosclerotic plaques or thrombi, as well as quantification of stenosis. Using PMCTA, small vascular lesions can be successfully detected; these include tiny aneurysms in the circle of Willis (**Fig. 17**) or posterior fossa (**Fig. 18**).

Furthermore, PMCTA is useful for localizing the bleeding source in most cases of vascular rupture, which is time-consuming or occasionally impossible during standard autopsy.[13-15]

9.4. Airway and thoracic diseases

Asphyxia refers to a condition that leads to impaired gas exchange, causing hypoxia and hypercapnia. Oxygen supply can be blocked at many stages (e.g., oxygen passage to lungs, delivery to tissues, and transport into the cell membrane).[48]

Choking is a mechanical type of asphyxia, which occurs when food materials or foreign objects block the throat or upper airway (**Fig. 19**). However, any other condition with the potential to block the airway can lead to choking; such conditions include soft tissue swelling with airway inflammation and infection, tumors in the oral cavity and laryngopharynx (**Figs. 20 and 21**)[49], and extrinsic compression by strangulation. Although deaths from choking are usually accidental and associated with food materials impacted in the airway, most victims have predisposing factors for choking such as old age, poor dentition, alcohol consumption, drug-related sedation, and neurological disease.[50-52] PMCT is also useful for pre-autopsy inspection of the tracheobronchial system to identify foreign materials and airway obstruction (**Fig. 22**). In cases where mechanical choking is suspected as a potential cause of death, PMCT can further assist pathologists in tailoring the dissection, with respect to guiding the identification of foreign materials and targeting lesions for histological sampling, thereby reducing the time and effort required for autopsy dissection.[15, 53]

Respiratory diseases are major causes of natural death and include lung infection, chronic obstructive disease, and lung cancer; these contributed to 9.0 million deaths (16% of total deaths) worldwide

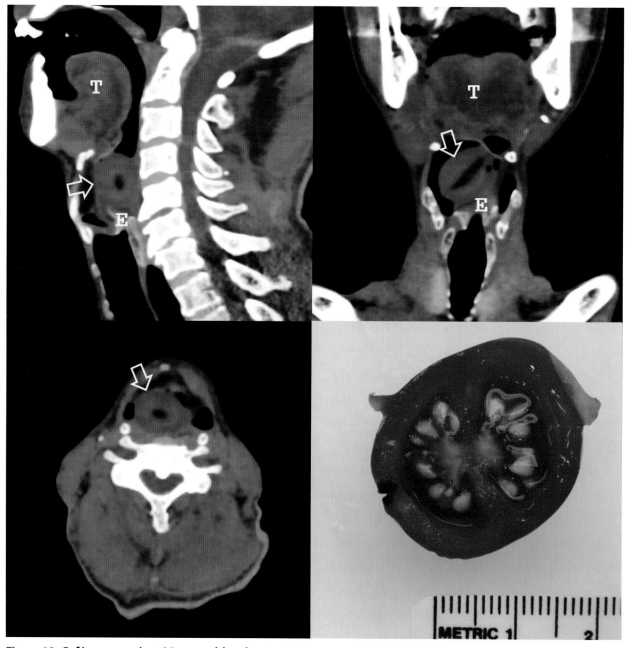

Figure 19. Café coronary in a 66-year-old male.

Sagittal (upper left), coronal (upper right), and axial (lower left) CT images show an oval-shaped foreign body (arrows) located between the root of the tongue and epiglottis, entirely blocking the oropharynx and leading to death from choking. A cherry tomato was removed from the oropharynx during autopsy and cut in half (lower right).
T: tongue, E: epiglottis.

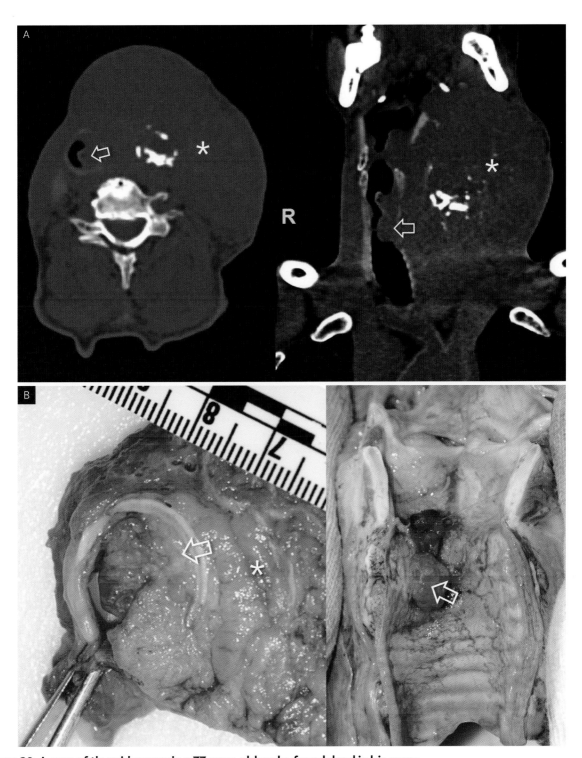

Figure 20. A case of thyroid cancer in a 77-year-old male, found dead in his room.

Postmortem CT axial (left) and coronal (right) images (A) show right-sided deviation of the trachea by a large thyroid tumor (*) and severe obstruction of the tracheal lumen by tumor invasion (arrow). Photographs of cut section (B) of the trachea in axial (left) and coronal (right) planes show tracheal invasion by the tumor and consequent luminal narrowing of the trachea.

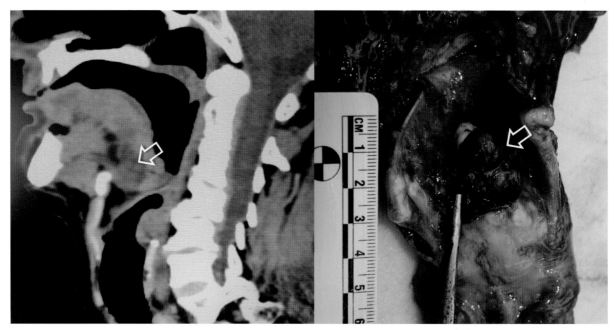

Figure 21. A case with epiglottis cyst in a 63-year-old male found dead in his bed.
Postmortem CT image (left) demonstrates a well-defined hypodense cyst with thin wall (arrow) at the lingual surface of the epiglottis measuring approximately 2×2 cm, which was identified as an epiglottic cyst (arrow in right) during autopsy dissection. Epithelial cysts of the larynx (commonly epiglottis) may produce sudden and unexpected death from asphyxia, although it is histologically benign and patients are sometimes asymptomatic (see Med Sci Law. 1995 Jan;35(1):72-4).

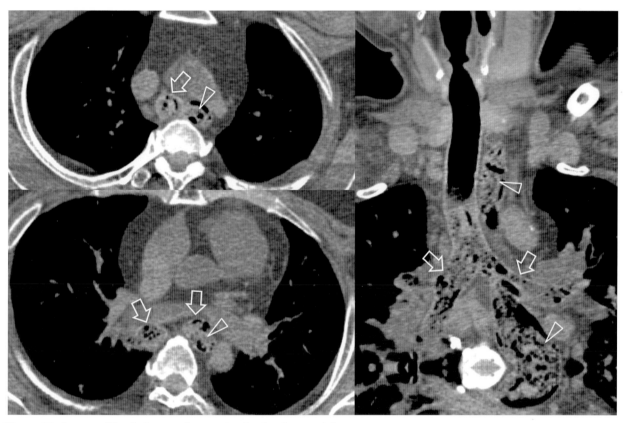

Figure 22. A case of fatal airway obstruction by food materials.

The tracheobronchial tree is completely filled with mottled soft tissue densities (arrows) in a coronal CT image, and the densities were identified as aspirated food material during autopsy. The food material (arrowheads) is also evident in the esophageal lumen.

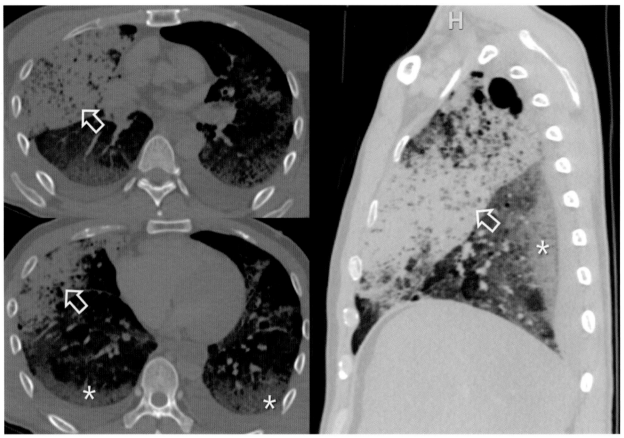

Figure 23. Postmortem CT of a case of suppurative pneumonia.
Axial (left upper and lower) and sagittal (right) images in lung window setting show a lobar distribution of consolidation in the right upper and lower lobes (arrows). CT images also show ground-glass opacities (*) with a well-defined horizontal border in the dependent position of both lower lobes, suggestive of postmortem hypostasis or sedimentation (livor mortis).

in 2016.[3] Although not typically associated with respiratory disease, sudden death may occur in cases with pulmonary thromboembolism; asthma-related bronchospasm and airway obstruction; and massive hemoptysis related to pulmonary tuberculosis, pneumonia, and tumors. Deaths from pneumonia are rarely subject to death investigation because death is often expected in severe cases in clinical settings. However, if the causative organism is highly virulent or if the victim's immune system is suppressed, a death investigation may be performed. PMCT

provides minimal insights regarding the suspected cause of death when it is attributed to respiratory infection (e.g., bacterial pneumonia). Patchy ill-defined and focal well-defined consolidation with pleural effusion are the typical CT findings of bronchopneumonia and lobar pneumonia, respectively (**Fig. 23**).[54] However, the diagnosis should be established microbiologically and histologically. Total or near-total opacification of the lungs may be present on PMCT in severe cases. Differentiation between consolidation of infectious or neoplastic origin, relative to

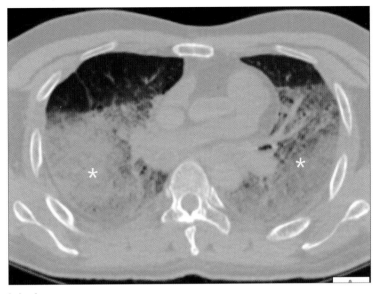

Figure 24. Hypostasis of the lungs.
Axial postmortem CT image shows gradually increasing density (*) from upper to lower dependent positions of the bilateral subpleural lungs in the lung window setting.

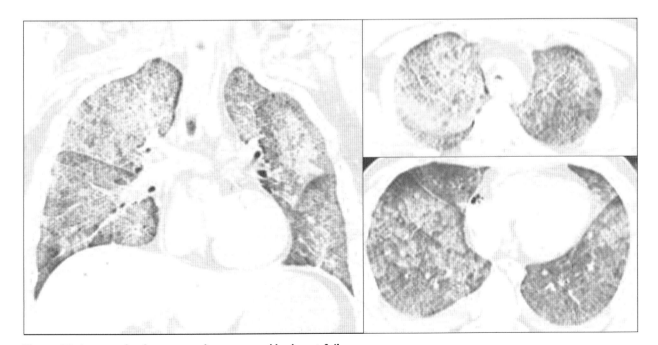

Figure 25. A case of pulmonary edema caused by heart failure.
Coronal (right) and axial (left upper and lower) images of postmortem CT show bilateral symmetrical ground-glass opacities and consolidations with inter- and intralobular septal thickenings, indicative of pulmonary edema rather than pneumonia or postmortem sedimentation.

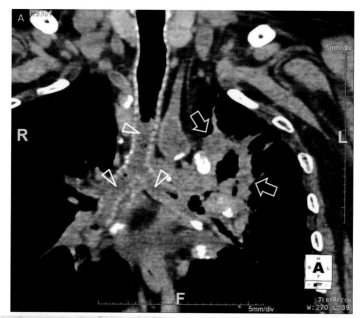

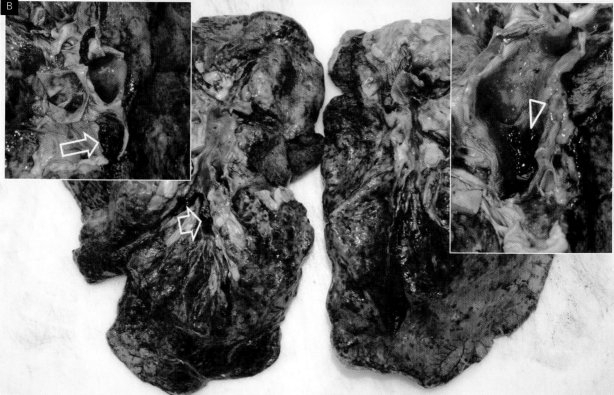

Figure 26. Hemoptysis due to lung cancer and blood aspiration into the airway in a 58-year-old male.

(A) Coronal CT image shows a cavitary lung mass (arrows) in the left perihilar area and blood (arrowheads) in the lumen of the trachea and bronchi, indicative of airway bleeding related to lung cancer. This lesion was identified as squamous cell carcinoma during histological examination. (B) Photograph of the pathologic specimen shows blood clots in the lobar bronchi in the magnified boxes (arrow in the right lung and arrowhead in the left lung), and a linear clot in the segmental bronchi of the right lung (short arrow).

hypostasis (livor mortis) in the dependent position, is occasionally difficult and may be impossible without histological examination. Hypostasis is the first postmortem finding identified on CT immediately after death, appearing as bilateral symmetrical ground-glass opacities in the dependent lung **(Fig. 24)**.

In contrast, patchy peribronchial consolidations with asymmetrical distribution may suggest abnormal pathological conditions, mostly involving pneumonia.[15] Postmortem CT imaging can also be used to screen for various pulmonary and mediastinal diseases that may be partly associated with death, or

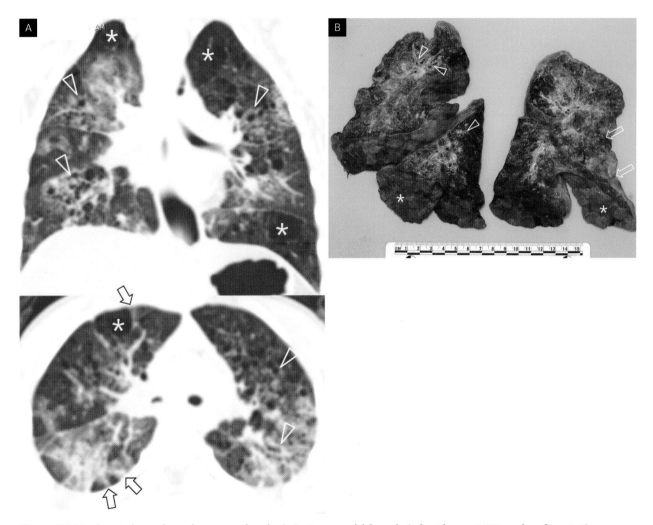

Figure 27. Moderate bronchopulmonary dysplasia in 6-year-old female infant born at 27 weeks of gestation.
(A) Transverse (upper) and coronal (lower) postmortem CT scans show regional air trappings (*), bronchial wall thickenings (arrowheads), subsegmental/segmental atelectasis, consolidation, and architectural distortion with parenchymal bands (arrows) in all segments of both upper and lower lobes. (B) Autopsy photography of the lungs shows diffuse thickening of the bronchial walls and alternating pattern of hyperexpanded and collapsed acini defined by irregular pseudofissures (arrows) and cobble stone appearance (*) of the pleural surface (see RadioGraphics 2005; 25:1047–1073).

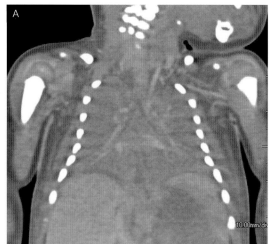

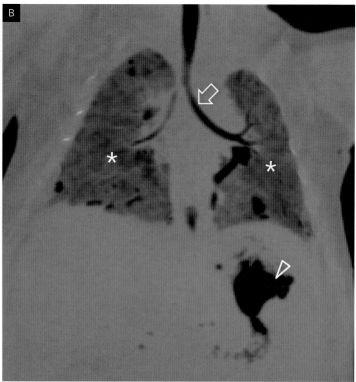

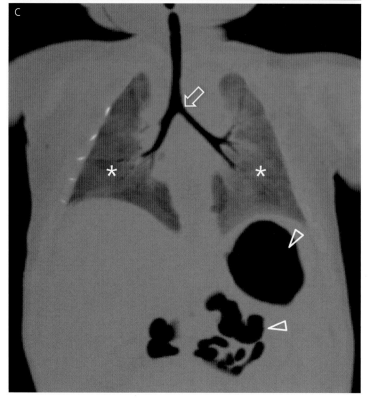

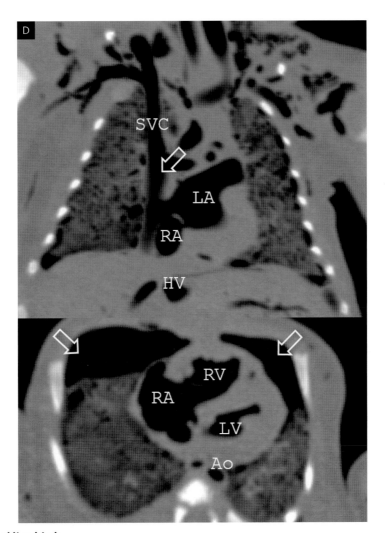

Figure 28. Stillbirth and live birth.
(A) Postmortem CT coronal multiplanar reformation image of a baby with intrauterine death. (B) Coronal minimum intensity projection image of a neonate found dead in a box abandoned in an apartment flowerbed. (C) Coronal minimum intensity projection image of a neonate. Emergency cesarean section was performed due to maternal uterine rupture and cardiopulmonary resuscitation (CPR) was carried out immediately after delivery to assist the newborn who did not breathe. (D) Coronal (upper) and axial (lower) image of a neonate acquired 7 days after birth on a toilet. To differentiate between live birth and stillbirth in a discarded newborn, the standard test (used in most death investigations) is the lung flotation test, occasionally including the stomach and duodenum. The air-containing lungs of a newborn who breathed at birth float in the water, while the lungs of a newborn who did not breathe are submerged. When determining whether a newborn experienced live birth or stillbirth, postmortem CT can be useful as an additional tool to the traditional flotation test to detect lung aeration, a sign of live birth. Using CT, the air in the lungs and stomach is clearly visible in a liveborn neonate, while a stillborn neonate does not have these signs. In a stillborn neonate (A), postmortem CT shows no air in the tracheobronchial tree and lungs. However, it demonstrates air in the lungs (*), tracheobronchial system (arrow), and stomach (arrowhead) (i.e., signs of live birth) in a liveborn neonate (B). As in the floatation test, care is needed when interpreting the finding of aerated lungs (*) and air in the gastrointestinal tract (arrowheads) in cases where CPR has been carried out (C) or in cases that show signs of putrefaction (D). In cases of putrefaction, the gases reportedly develop in the liver at a similar rate to that in lung tissue, and postmortem CT can be used to detect the presence or absence of putrefactive gas in the body structures such as large vessels (arrow in upper), cardiac chambers, and body cavities (arrows in lower). SVC: superior vena cava, LA: left atrium, RA: right atrium, LV: left atrium, HV: hepatic vein, Ao: Aorta

to find indications of signs of vitality after specific events **(Fig. 25-28)**.

Pulmonary thromboembolism is a leading cause of natural death frequently encountered in forensic death investigations. Although it cannot be diagnosed with postmortem CT **(Fig. 29)**, it can be identified as an intraluminal filling defect after antegrade contrast injection into the right heart and pulmonary arteries through the femoral vein **(Fig. 30)**.

However, right heart and segmental to subsegmental pulmonary arteries are the most common structures where postmortem clotting tends to develop, especially in cases with a longstanding agonal period.[55, 56] Therefore, any filling defects in these pulmonary arterial branches could be associated with either antemortem thromboembolus or postmortem

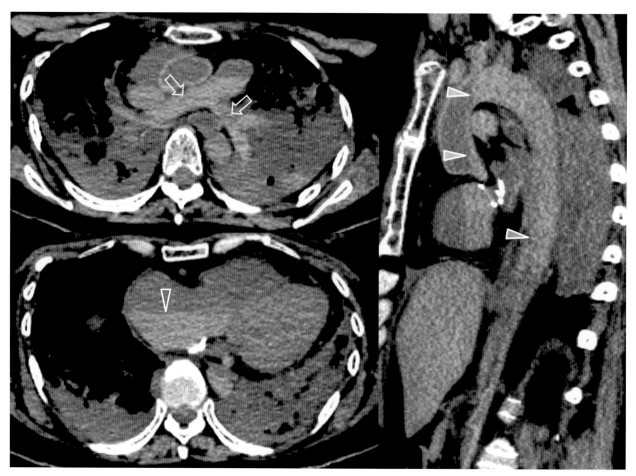

Figure 29. Postmortem CT of a case of pulmonary thromboembolism.
Axial (left upper and lower) and sagittal images (right). Axial images at the level of the pulmonary and main pulmonary arteries show a dense material present in both main pulmonary arteries, which was identified as pulmonary thromboembolism. Occasionally, pulmonary thromboembolism can exhibit high density as in this case, but it is difficult to distinguish from postmortem hemoconcentration, commonly found in large vessels and cardiac chambers as shown in the right atrium (arrowhead in left lower) and aorta (white-filled arrowheads in right). See Chapter 12 for more information regarding hemoconcentration.

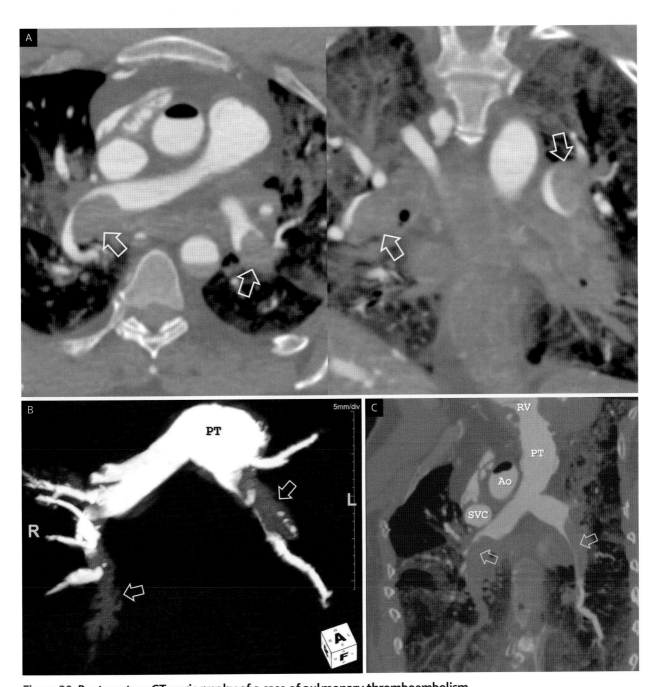

Figure 30. Postmortem CT angiography of a case of pulmonary thromboembolism.
(A) Axial (left upper and lower) and coronal (right) multiplanar images show irregular contrast filling defects in the right (arrows) and left (arrowheads) pulmonary arteries. (B) Maximum intensity projection and (C) medial axis reformation images provide a better understanding of the spatial relationship between pulmonary arteries and thrombi. Advanced postprocessing techniques can be used to condense diagnostic information from various angles and perspectives, and can aid in identifying lesions in a more intuitive manner.

clotting. However, elongated contrast defects in the pulmonary trunk and main pulmonary arteries are reportedly indicative of thromboembolism, rather than postmortem clots.[13] Nevertheless, pulmonary thromboembolism should be diagnosed based on histological analysis of suspected thromboembolic materials obtained from CT-guided biopsy or autopsy dissection.[13, 15, 56]

9.5. Intraabdominal diseases

Deaths from natural intra-abdominal pathologies are usually not subject to forensic death investigation. However, massive bleeding from the gastrointestinal tract, peritoneal cavity, and extraperitoneal structures may be causes of sudden death. Such fatal hemorrhage of the digestive tract is caused by peptic ulcers, ruptured varices, or tumors. In contrast, intra and retroperitoneal hemorrhages are associated with various underlying pathologies: aneurysmal rupture of the aorta (**Fig. 31**) and its smaller visceral branches; rupture of the liver and spleen secondary to tumors, infection, or other hematological disorders; and gynecological conditions such as rupture of an ovarian cyst and ectopic pregnancy.[57]

Acute bleeding appears hyperdense on noncontrast CT, and hyperdense blood on PMCT indicates acute stage of hemorrhage at the time of death. As described earlier, normal physiological evolution of hemoglobin ceases immediately after death. Therefore, CT density of hemorrhage reflects the age of hemorrhagic blood at the time of death, independently of the time since death. Hemorrhagic blood

in the peritoneal cavity tends to spread into various dependent spaces, such as the hepatorenal space, paracolic gutters, rectouterine pouch in females, and rectovesical space in males. However, in most cases, hemorrhagic blood collects near the bleeding source at early initiation of bleeding with the sentinel clot sign (high-density fluid surrounding the bleeding organ) on nonenhanced CT (**Fig. 32**).[58] The sentinel clot sign can be used to suggest potential causes of acute bleeding in the postmortem setting. However, PMCTA can pinpoint the site of rupture by direct visualization of contrast leakage through the defect, helping to suggest vascular rupture as a cause of death. PMCT can detect gaseous distention of bowel loops (**Fig. 33**). In cases of hollow viscus perforation, PMCT can help to detect various amounts of free intra-abdominal gas collection, if any (**Fig. 34**). Although PMCT can also depict the outer contours of intra-abdominal solid organs, However, there are potential limitations in the evaluation of internal structures of these organs due to its inherently low tissue contrast. PMCTA shows a variable degree of parenchymal enhancement, depending on the vascularity of each organ and type of postmortem contrast agents. Contrast enhancement of respective organs helps to identify parenchymal abnormalities (e.g., tumors or other space-occupying lesions), providing better contrast between space-occupying pathologies and surrounding normal parenchyma. Furthermore, contrast enhancement helps to distinguish soft tissue structures with similar densities (e.g., enlarged lymph nodes from adjacent organs and blood vessels) (**Fig. 35**).[15]

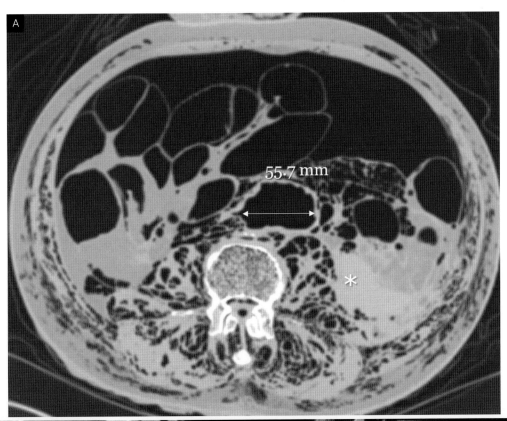

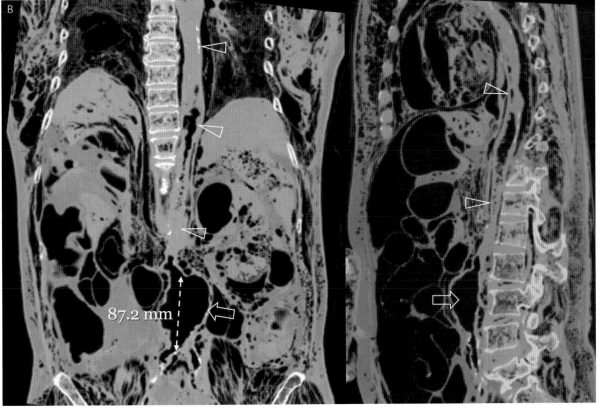

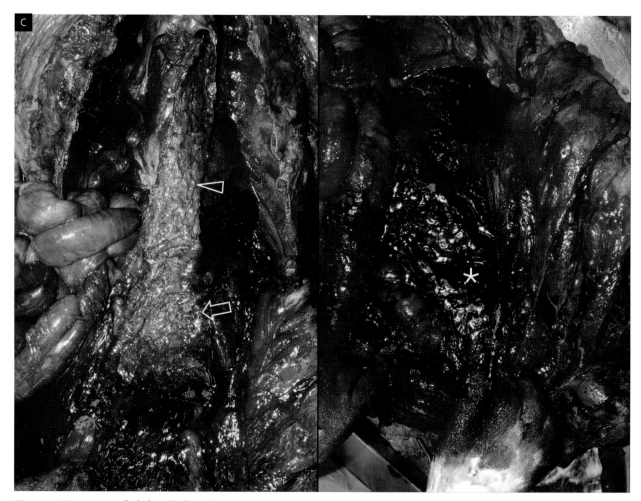

Figure 31. Rupture of abdominal aortic aneurysm.
(A) Axial image of postmortem CT of a highly decomposed case shows high-density intra-abdominal hemorrhage (*) and focal dilatation (double-headed arrows) of the aorta containing putrefactive gas. (B) Coronal (left) and sagittal (right) images show thoracoabdominal aorta with focal dilatation arrows of the gas-filled lower abdominal aorta and extensive gas collection in all tissue planes, as well as organ collapse due to decomposition (see Chapter 12 for the details of postmortem changes). Note the air-containing collapsed thoracic aorta (arrowheads). (C) Autopsy photographs show the abdominal aorta (arrowhead) and focal rupture of the dilatated aorta (arrow) and periaortic hematoma (*).

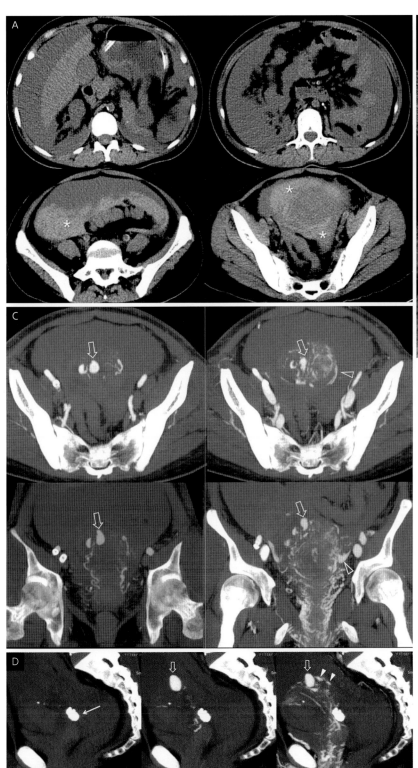

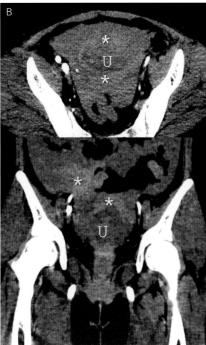

Figure 32. A 26-year-old female with fatal hemorrhage from a ruptured uterine tumor.

Antemortem axial CT images (A) show extensive fluid collection in the abdominal cavity with a high-density fluid (*) surrounding the uterus in the pelvic cavity, indicating acute hemorrhage from the uterus as a source of hemorrhagic blood (sentinel clot sign). In B, postmortem coronal (upper) and axial (lower) images also depict a comparatively high-density hemorrhage (*) near the uterus (sentinel clot sign). (C) After arterial (left) and subsequent venous contrast injection (right), axial (upper row) and coronal (lower row) images of postmortem CT demonstrate multiple arterial aneurysms (arrows) and contrast leakage from dilated venous structures (arrowheads). Sagittal images (D) of postmortem CT before contrast enhancement (left), after arterial injection (middle), and subsequent venous injection (right) demonstrate arterial aneurysm (arrows), dilated venous structures (arrowheads), and calcification (long arrow), respectively. Autopsy confirmed rupture of the uterus associated with the uterine angiomyoma. U: uterus.

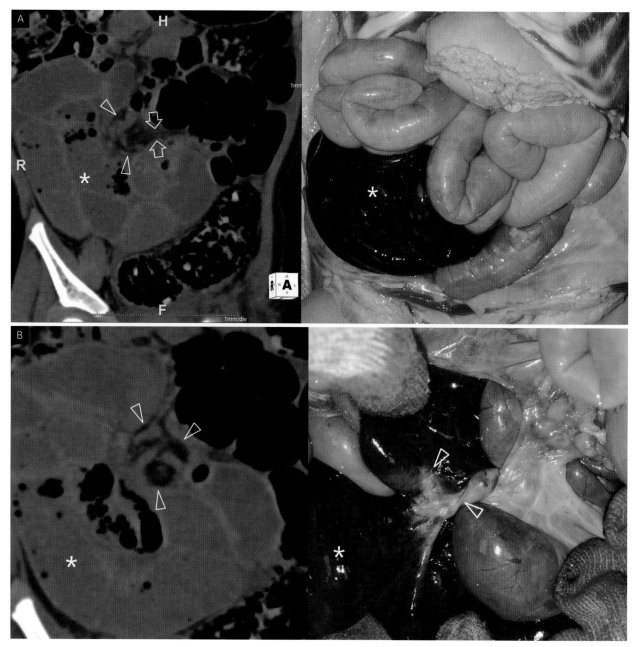

Figure 33. A 1-year-old baby with mesenteric volvulus and small bowel obstruction.

(A) Postmortem CT images (left) reconstructed in the oblique coronal plane, perpendicular to mesenteric vessel (arrows) and surrounding soft tissue (arrowheads) whirling, shows fluid-distended (*) and gas-distended bowel loops in the right lower and left upper abdomen, respectively. Autopsy photograph (right) shows dark purple discoloration of fluid-distended bowel loops with necrotic changes (*). (B) Oblique sagittal image (left) reconstructed in the vertical planes depicts whirling (arrowheads) of mesenteric vessels, fat, and soft tissues surrounded by twisted and distended small bowel loops (*). Autopsy photograph (right) shows twisted mesentery (arrowheads) and bowel loops with necrotic changes with dark purple discoloration (*).

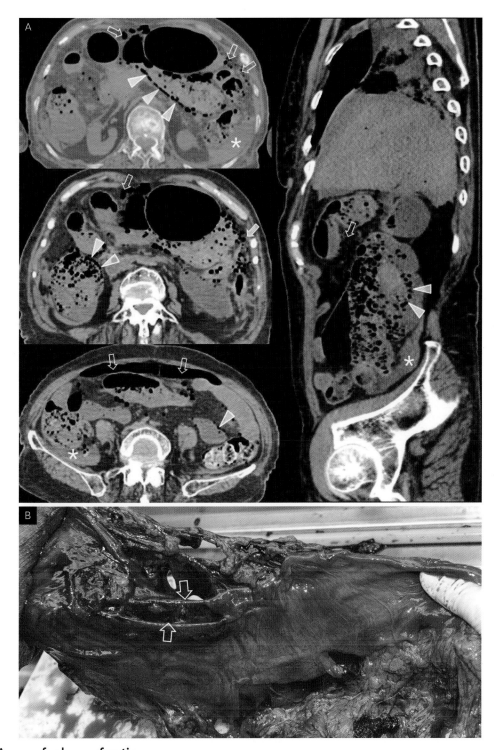

Figure 34. A case of colon perforation.

(A) Axial (left row) and sagittal (right) images of postmortem CT demonstrate multiple air densities along the large bowel walls (arrowheads); the images also show free air collection in the non-dependent position of the peritoneal cavity (arrow) and widely spread small air densities (arrowheads) in the mesentery and omental fat, indicative of necrotizing enterocolitis and bowel perforation. (B) Autopsy photograph shows the defect (arrows) in the wall of the ascending colon.

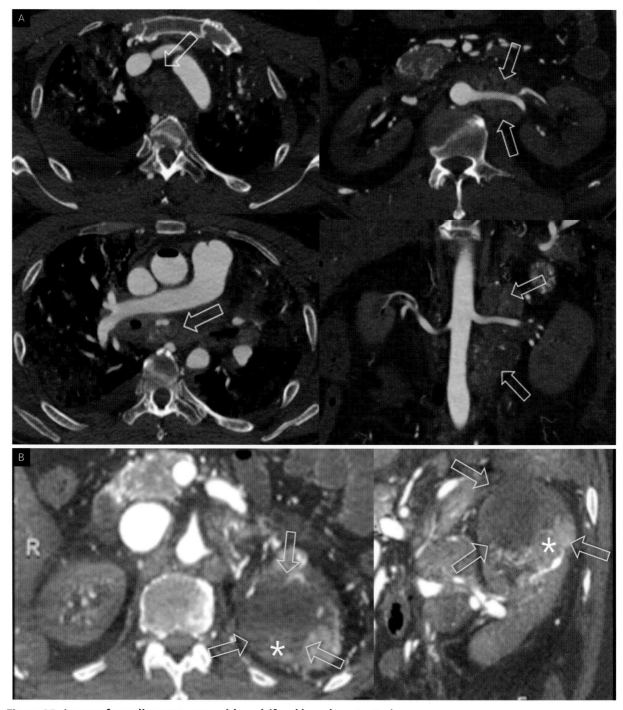

Figure 35. A case of a malignant tumor with multifocal lymph metastasis.

(A) Postmortem CT angiography shows enlarged lymph nodes at mediastinum (left upper and lower axial images) and periaortic area adjacent to the renal artery (right upper axial and lower coronal images). (B) Contrast enhancement helps to identify renal parenchymal abnormalities, providing better contrast between surrounding normal parenchyma and tumor (outlined by arrows) on axial (left) and coronal (right) images; these manifestations were subsequently identified as renal cell carcinoma during histological examination. Note the presence of heterogenous contrast enhancement of the tumor with stronger peripheral enhancement (*) and less central enhancement, reflecting internal vascularity within the tumor.

9.6. Summary

In cases of natural death, PMCT can be used to detect fatal hemorrhages that could have led to death (e.g., intracerebral hemorrhage and hemopericardium) and identify abnormal gas accumulations (e.g., air embolism and free air in the body cavity). Furthermore, PMCTA allows visualization of the arterial and venous systems, along with localization of the sites of rupture or occlusion. Finally, PMCT and PMCTA play useful roles in pre-autopsy screening for potential causes of death, guiding subsequent dissection for the visual demonstration of lesions that may be difficult or impossible to identify by autopsy dissection alone.

Reference

1   Oehmichen M, Meissner C. Natural death. Gerontology. 2000; 46(2):105-10. doi: 10.1159/000022143.

2   Janssen W..[Definition and reporting of unnatural death in the medical field] Beitrage zur gerichtlichen Medizin. 1979;37:105-8.

3   World Health Oranization: The top 10 causes of death. https://www.who.int/en/news-room/fact-sheets/detail/the-top-10-causes-of-death (2018). Accessed 05 July 2019.

4   Levy A, Harcke HJ. Natural death. In: Angela D. Levy HTH, editor. Essentials of forensic imaging: A text atlas. Boca Raton, FL: CRC Press; 2011. p. 217-34.

5   Koehler S. Death Investigation. In: Freeman M, Zeegers M, editors. Forensic Epidemiology Principles and Practice. London, UK: Elsevier Inc.; 2016. p. 179-99.

6   Biorck G, Wikland B. "Sudden death"--what are we talking about? Circulation. 1972;45(2):256-8. doi: 10.1161/01.cir.45.2.256.

7   La Russa R, Catalano C, Di Sanzo M, Scopetti M, Gatto V, Santurro A, et al. Postmortem computed tomography angiography (PMCTA) and traditional autopsy in cases of sudden cardiac death due to coronary artery disease: a systematic review and meta-analysis. La Radiologia medica. 2019;124(2):109-17. doi: 10.1007/s11547-018-0943-y.

8   Virmani R, Burke AP, Farb A. Sudden cardiac death. Cardiovascular pathology : the official journal of the Society for Cardiovascular Pathology. 2001;10(5):211-8.

9   McElwee SK, Velasco A, Doppalapudi H. Mechanisms of sudden cardiac death. Journal of nuclear cardiology: official publication of the American Society of Nuclear Cardiology. 2016;23(6):1368-79. doi: 10.1007/s12350-016-0600-6.

10 Michaud K, Grabherr S, Doenz F, Mangin P. Evaluation of post-mortem MDCT and MDCT-angiography for the investigation of sudden cardiac death related to atherosclerotic coronary artery disease. The international journal of cardiovascular imaging. 2012;28(7): 1807-22. doi: 10.1007/s10554-012-0012-x.

11 Chugh SS, Reinier K, Teodorescu C, Evanado A, Kehr E, Al Samara M, et al. Epidemiology of sudden cardiac death: clinical and research implications. Progress in cardiovascular diseases. 2008;51(3):213-28. doi: 10.1016/j.pcad.2008.06.003.

12 Risgaard B, Lynge TH, Wissenberg M, Jabbari R, Glinge C, Gislason GH, et al. Risk factors and causes of sudden noncardiac death: A nationwide cohort study in Denmark. Heart rhythm. 2015;12(5):968-74. doi: 10.1016/j.hrthm.2015.01.024.

13 Ross SG, Bolliger SA, Ampanozi G, Oesterhelweg L, Thali MJ, Flach PM. Postmortem CT angiography: capabilities and limitations in traumatic and natural causes of death. Radiographics : a review publication of the Radiological Society of North America, Inc. 2014; 34(3):830-46. doi: 10.1148/rg.343115169.

14 Grabherr S, Grimm J, Dominguez A, Vanhaebost J, Mangin P. Advances in post-mortem CT-angiography. The British journal of radiology. 2014;87(1036):20130488. doi: 10.1259/bjr.20130488.

15 Lee H, Lee S, Cha JG, Baek T, Yang KM. Postmortem Computed Tomography and Computed Tomography Angiography: Cardiothoracic Imaging Applications in Forensic Medicine. Journal of thoracic imaging. 2019. doi: 10.1097/rti.0000000000000398.

16 Maron BJ, Epstein SE, Roberts WC. Causes of sudden death in competitive athletes. Journal of the American College of Cardiology. 1986;7(1):204-14.

17 Morgan B, Biggs MJ, Barber J, Raj V, Amoroso J, Hollingbury FE, et al. Accuracy of targeted post-mortem computed tomography coronary angiography compared to assessment of serial histological sections. International journal of legal medicine. 2013;127(4):809-17. doi: 10.1007/s00414-012-0790-7.

18 Huikuri HV, Castellanos A, Myerburg RJ. Sudden death due to

cardiac arrhythmias. The New England journal of medicine. 2001; 345(20):1473-82. doi: 10.1056/NEJMra000650.

19   Polacco M, Sedati P, Arena V, Pascali VL, Zobel BB, Oliva A, et al. Visualization of myocardial infarction by post-mortem single-organ coronary computed tomography: a feasibility study. International journal of legal medicine. 2015;129(3):517-24. doi: 10.1007/s00414-014-1085-y.

20   Palmiere C, Lobrinus JA, Mangin P, Grabherr S. Detection of coronary thrombosis after multi-phase postmortem CT-angiography. Legal medicine (Tokyo, Japan). 2013;15(1):12-8. doi: 10.1016/j.legalmed.2012.08.005.

21   Rumberger JA, Simons DB, Fitzpatrick LA, Sheedy PF, Schwartz RS. Coronary artery calcium area by electron-beam computed tomography and coronary atherosclerotic plaque area. A histopathologic correlative study. Circulation. 1995;92(8):2157-62. doi: 10. 1161/01.cir.92.8.2157.

22   Leontiev O, Dubinsky TJ. CT-based calcium scoring to screen for coronary artery disease: why aren't we there yet? AJR American journal of roentgenology. 2007;189(5):1061-3. doi: 10.2214/ajr.07.2591.

23   Oudkerk M, Stillman AE, Halliburton SS, Kalender WA, Mohlenkamp S, McCollough CH, et al. Coronary artery calcium screening: current status and recommendations from the European Society of Cardiac Radiology and North American Society for Cardiovascular Imaging. The international journal of cardiovascular imaging. 2008;24(6):645-71. doi: 10.1007/s10554-008-9319-z.

24   Mantovani V, Vanoli D, Chelazzi P, Lepore V, Ferrarese S, Sala A. Post-infarction cardiac rupture: surgical treatment. European journal of cardio-thoracic surgery : official journal of the European Association for Cardio-thoracic Surgery. 2002;22(5):777-80. doi: 10.1016/s1010-7940(02)00485-2.

25   Figueras J, Alcalde O, Barrabes JA, Serra V, Alguersuari J, Cortadellas J, et al. Changes in hospital mortality rates in 425 patients with acute ST-elevation myocardial infarction and cardiac rupture over a 30-year period. Circulation. 2008;118(25):2783-9. doi: 10.1161/circulationaha.108.776690.

26   Filograna L, Thali MJ, Marchetti D. Forensic relevance of postmortem CT imaging of the haemopericardium in determining the cause of death. Legal medicine (Tokyo, Japan). 2014;16(5):247-51. doi: 10.1016/j.legalmed.2014.05.005.

27   Shiotani S, Watanabe K, Kohno M, Ohashi N, Yamazaki K, Nakayama H. Postmortem computed tomographic (PMCT) findings of pericardial effusion due to acute aortic dissection. Radiation medicine. 2004;22(6):405-7.

28   Corvera JS. Acute aortic syndrome. Annals of cardiothoracic surgery. 2016;5(3):188-93. doi: 10.21037/acs.2016.04.05.

29   Bossone E, LaBounty TM, Eagle KA. Acute aortic syndromes: diagnosis and management, an update. European heart journal. 2018; 39(9):739-49d. doi: 10.1093/eurheartj/ehx319.

30   Lempel JK, Frazier AA, Jeudy J, Kligerman SJ, Schultz R, Ninalowo HA, et al. Aortic arch dissection: a controversy of classification. Radiology. 2014;271(3):848-55. doi: 10.1148/radiol.14131457.

31   Johnston KW, Rutherford RB, Tilson MD, Shah DM, Hollier L, Stanley JC. Suggested standards for reporting on arterial aneurysms. Subcommittee on Reporting Standards for Arterial Aneurysms, Ad Hoc Committee on Reporting Standards, Society for Vascular Surgery and North American Chapter, International Society for Cardiovascular Surgery. Journal of vascular surgery. 1991;13(3):452-8.

32   Aggarwal S, Qamar A, Sharma V, Sharma A. Abdominal aortic aneurysm: A comprehensive review. Experimental and clinical cardiology. 2011;16(1):11-5.

33   Munden RF, Carter BW, Chiles C, MacMahon H, Black WC, Ko JP, et al. Managing Incidental Findings on Thoracic CT: Mediastinal and Cardiovascular Findings. A White Paper of the ACR Incidental Findings Committee. Journal of the American College of Radiology : JACR. 2018;15(8):1087-96. doi: 10.1016/j.jacr.2018.04.029.

34   McComb BL, Munden RF, Duan F, Jain AA, Tuite C, Chiles C. Normative reference values of thoracic aortic diameter in American College of Radiology Imaging Network (ACRIN 6654) arm of National Lung Screening Trial. Clinical imaging. 2016;40(5):936-43. doi: 10.1016/j.clinimag.2016.04.013.

35   Johnson W, Onuma O, Owolabi M, Sachdev S. Stroke: a global response is needed. Bulletin of the World Health Organization. 2016;94(9):634-a. doi: 10.2471/blt.16.181636.

36   Owolabi MO, Akarolo-Anthony S, Akinyemi R, Arnett D, Gebregziabher M, Jenkins C, et al. The burden of stroke in Africa: a glance at the present and a glimpse into the future. Cardiovascular journal of Africa. 2015;26(2 Suppl 1):S27-38. doi: 10.5830/cvja-2015-038.

37   Lloyd-Jones D, Adams R, Carnethon M, De Simone G, Ferguson TB, Flegal K, et al. Heart disease and stroke statistics--2009 update: a report from the American Heart Association Statistics Committee and Stroke Statistics Subcommittee. Circulation. 2009;119(3):480-6. doi: 10.1161/circulationaha.108.191259.

38   Runchey S, McGee S. Does this patient have a hemorrhagic stroke?: clinical findings distinguishing hemorrhagic stroke from ischemic stroke. Jama. 2010;303(22):2280-6. doi: 10.1001/jama.2010.754.

39   Musuka TD, Wilton SB, Traboulsi M, Hill MD. Diagnosis and management of acute ischemic stroke: speed is critical. CMAJ : Canadian Medical Association journal = journal de l'Association medicale canadienne. 2015;187(12):887-93. doi: 10.1503/cmaj.140355.

40   Dennis MS, Burn JP, Sandercock PA, Bamford JM, Wade DT, Warlow CP. Long-term survival after first-ever stroke: the Oxfordshire Community Stroke Project. Stroke. 1993;24(6):796-800.

41   Sacco RL, Wolf PA, Kannel WB, McNamara PM. Survival and recur-

rence following stroke. The Framingham study. Stroke. 1982;13(3):290-5.

42   Andersen KK, Olsen TS, Dehlendorff C, Kammersgaard LP. Hemorrhagic and ischemic strokes compared: stroke severity, mortality, and risk factors. Stroke. 2009;40(6):2068-72. doi: 10.1161/strokeaha. 108.540112.

43   Mansour TR, Alam Y, Dahbour L, Alnemari A, Jumaa M, Schroeder JL. Streptococcus Mutans: A Potential Risk Factor in Recurrent Hemorrhagic Stroke. Cureus. 2017;9(5):e1264. doi: 10.7759/cureus.1264.

44   Smith AB, Lattin GE, Jr., Berran P, Harcke HT. Common and expected postmortem CT observations involving the brain: mimics of antemortem pathology. AJNR American journal of neuroradiology. 2012;33(7):1387-91. doi: 10.3174/ajnr.A2966.

45   Ishida M, Gonoi W, Okuma H, Shirota G, Shintani Y, Abe H, et al. Common Postmortem Computed Tomography Findings Following Atraumatic Death: Differentiation between Normal Postmortem Changes and Pathologic Lesions. Korean journal of radiology. 2015; 16(4):798-809. doi: 10.3348/kjr.2015.16.4.798.

46   Parizel PM, Makkat S, Van Miert E, Van Goethem JW, van den Hauwe L, De Schepper AM. Intracranial hemorrhage: principles of CT and MRI interpretation. European radiology. 2001;11(9):1770-83. doi: 10.1007/s003300000800.

47   Ruder TD ZW, Hatch GM, Ross S, Ampanozi G, Thali MJ, Flach PM. Still frame from the hour of death - Acute intracerebral hemorrhage on post-mortem computed tomography in a decomposed corpse. Journal of Forensic Radiology and Imaging. 2013;1:73-6.

48   Byard R. Asphyxia: Pathological Features. In: Payne-James J, Byard R, editors. Encyclopedia of Forensic and Legal Medicine. 2nd ed. Amsterdam, Netherlands: Elsevier Inc.; 2016. p. 252-60.

49   Dada MA. Laryngeal cyst and sudden death. Medicine, science, and the law. 1995;35(1):72-4. doi: 10.1177/002580249503500114.

50   Wick R, Gilbert JD, Byard RW. Cafe coronary syndrome-fatal choking on food: an autopsy approach. Journal of clinical forensic medicine. 2006;13(3):135-8. doi: 10.1016/j.jcfm.2005.10.007.

51   Mittleman RE, Wetli CV. The fatal cafe coronary. Foreign-body airway obstruction. Jama. 1982;247(9):1285-8.

52   Iino M, O'Donnell C. Postmortem computed tomography findings of upper airway obstruction by food. Journal of forensic sciences. 2010;55(5):1251-8. doi: 10.1111/j.1556-4029.2010.01430.x.

53   Grabherr S, Heinemann A, Vogel H, Rutty G, Morgan B, Wozniak K, et al. Postmortem CT Angiography Compared with Autopsy: A Forensic Multicenter Study. Radiology. 2018;288(1):270-6. doi: 10.1148/radiol.2018170559.

54   Franquet T. Imaging of pulmonary viral pneumonia. Radiology. 2011;260(1):18-39. doi: 10.1148/radiol.11092149.

55   Ross SG, Thali MJ, Bolliger S, Germerott T, Ruder TD, Flach PM. Sudden death after chest pain: feasibility of virtual autopsy with postmortem CT angiography and biopsy. Radiology. 2012;264(1): 250-9. doi: 10.1148/radiol.12092415.

56   Bruguier C, Mosimann PJ, Vaucher P, Uské A, Doenz F, Jackowski C, et al. Multi-phase postmortem CT angiography: recognizing technique-related artefacts and pitfalls. International journal of legal medicine. 2013;127(3):639-52. doi: 10.1007/s00414-013-0840-9.

57   Lubner M, Menias C, Rucker C, Bhalla S, Peterson CM, Wang L, et al. Blood in the belly: CT findings of hemoperitoneum. Radiographics: a review publication of the Radiological Society of North America, Inc. 2007;27(1):109-25. doi: 10.1148/rg.271065042.

58   Orwig D, Federle MP. Localized clotted blood as evidence of visceral trauma on CT: the sentinel clot sign. AJR American journal of roentgenology. 1989;153(4):747-9. doi: 10.2214/ajr.153.4.747.

Chapter 10

Death with medicolegal issues

The past can hurt.
But, you can either run from it or learn from it.
− The Lion King

Postmortem CT (PMCT) has a wide range of forensic applications, including the investigation of medical interventions with fatal consequences. There has been an increasing number of reports describing the advantages of PMCT in detecting medical treatment errors.[1-4] Currently, many forensic institutions worldwide have incorporated PMCT as an integral part of the standard procedure for investigations of periprocedural deaths or unexpected deaths of hospitalized patients (Figs. 1-4).

The autopsy can be effectively guided by PMCT for the exact location of medical devices before opening the body in situations that involve a risk of repositioning such devices, particularly in cases with fatal outcomes caused by misplaced catheters, guidewires, and drainage tubes.[1] Although PMCT is useful for detecting internal hemorrhage less accessible to conventional dissection, PMCT angiography (PMCTA) is required to identify the source of bleeding and document major vascular patency after open vascular surgery and percutaneous endovascular interven-

tions (Figs. 5-8).[2, 5, 6]

According to a recent study regarding the potential role of CT examinations in assessing unexpected deaths of hospitalized patients, the addition of angiography improves the diagnostic performance of PMCT for detecting cardiovascular disease to the point where it can serve as a useful alternative in the absence of traditional autopsy.[4]

In contrast to trauma cases, medical malpractice cases more often involve bleeding sources in small arteries and veins, potentially without recognizable vascular defects. In those cases, PMCT often pinpoints the site of small-vessel bleeding, which is a time-consuming or impossible task during standard autopsy.[2, 7] Because contrast agent is injected into arterial and venous systems separately, PMCTA distinguishes the bleeding from arterial and venous sources, using both water and lipid-soluble agents.[8, 9] The amount of contrast leakage into body spaces often depends on the severity of vascular injury. However, this assumption may not be correct in soft

140

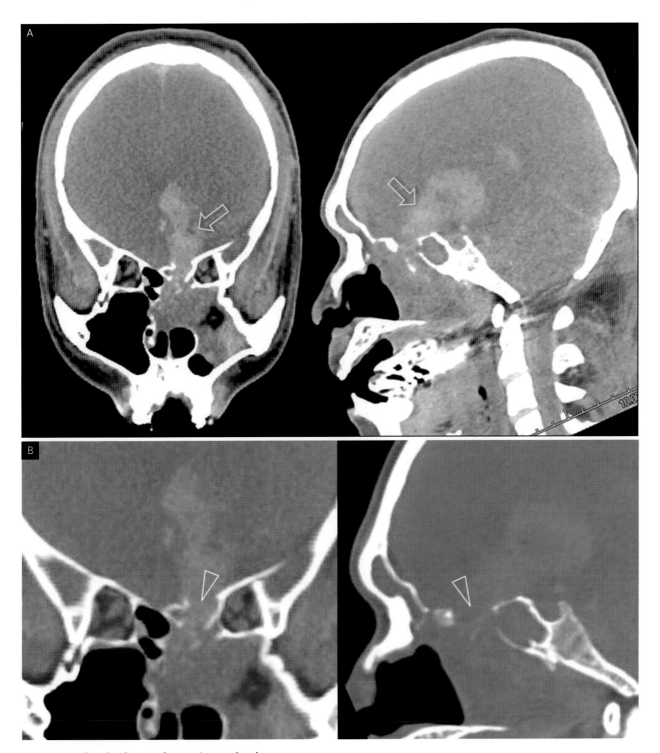

Figure 1. A death after endoscopic nasal polypectomy.
A 38-year-old male died of intracerebral hemorrhage and related complications after endoscopic nasal polypectomy for the treatment of nasal polyposis. (A) Oblique axial (left) and coronal (right) images of postmortem CT show intracranial hemorrhage (arrows) in the frontal lobe. (B) Images with bone window setting show destruction of the lamina papyracea (arrowheads).

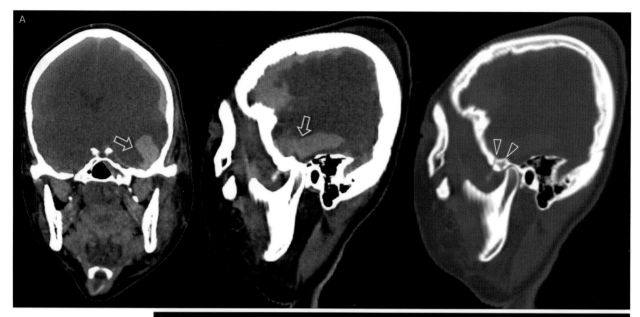

Figure 2. A death after zygoma reduction surgery.

A 27-year-old female died of intracerebral hemorrhage during zygoma reduction surgery. (A) Coronal (left) and parasagittal (middle) images of postmortem CT show intracerebral hemorrhage (arrows) in the left temporal lobe and subdural hemorrhage, as well as two sharp bony cuts in the temporal bone (arrowheads in right). Axial multiplanar reconstruction image in bone window setting (left) and maximum intensity projection image (right) in (B) and three-dimensional volume-rendered image (left in C) show two surgical saw blade marks (arrowheads) on the temporal bone, which was confirmed during autopsy dissection (right in C).

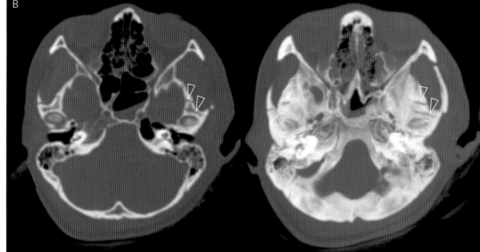

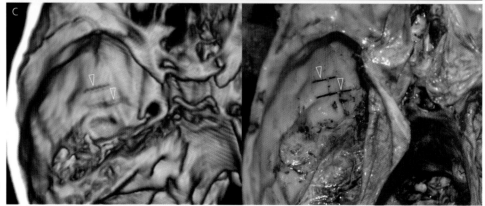

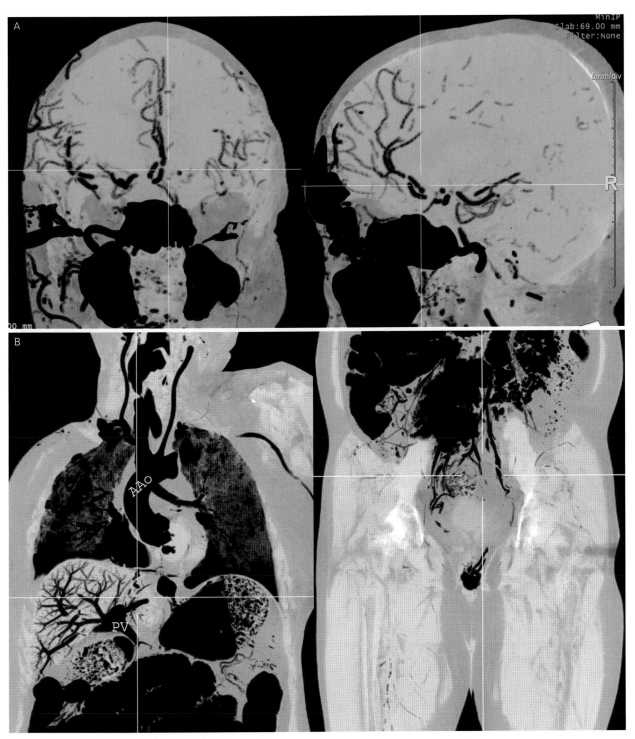

Figure 3. A case of death after intravenous injection of hydrogen-rich saline as an antioxidant.
Minimal intensity reconstruction images of postmortem CT show extensive systemic air embolism of cerebral arteries (A);
they also depict air in cardiac chambers, portal vein, and peripheral vessels (B).

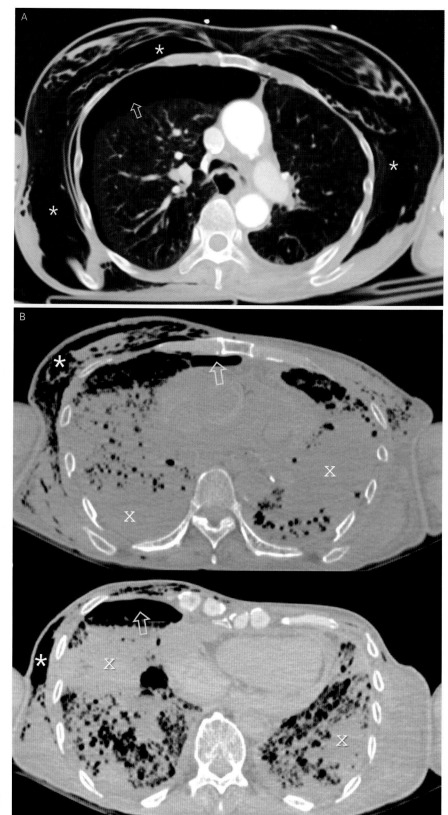

Figure 4. Acupuncture-related massive pneumothorax.

A 73-year-old male developed pneumothorax after acupuncture needles were inserted in his back. He was admitted to the hospital but died of pneumothorax-related complications including pneumonia. (A) Axial image of antemortem CT shows the right-sided pneumothorax (arrow) and bilateral extensive chest wall emphysema (*).
(B) Axial images of postmortem CT demonstrate localized right-sided pneumothorax (arrow) and chest wall emphysema (*). Note the presence of newly developed pneumonic consolidation (x) on both lower lobes during the course of treatment.

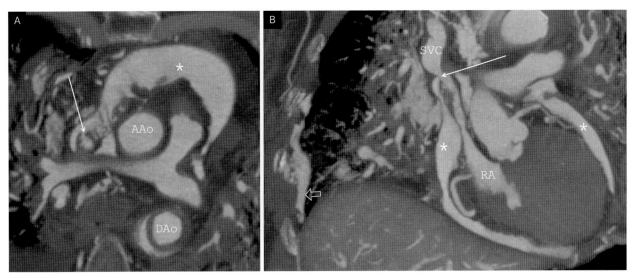

Figure 5. Rupture of the superior vena cava after endovascular intervention.
Oblique axial (A) and coronal (B) images of postmortem CT angiography show contrast leakage into the pericardial cavity (*) through an anterior wall defect of the superior vena cava (long arrows). Note the presence of rib fracture and hemorrhage into anterior chest wall (arrow in B) associated with cardiopulmonary resuscitation. AAo: ascending aorta, DAo: descending aorta, RA: right atrium.

tissue, particularly when antemortem and postmortem hematomas have become sufficiently enlarged to produce a compression effect on surrounding tissue.[1] Although PMCTA serves as an effective tool, particularly in the detection of bleeding source and identification of vessel luminal patency, there remain potential sources of errors in diagnosis solely based on CT examination.[9] For example, although filling defects in pulmonary arteries are clearly demonstrated after contrast filling, the differentiation of antemortem thromboembolism and postmortem clotting requires histological analysis of thromboembolic materials. The diagnosis of myocardial infarction requires histopathological examination performed during autopsy, and some persistent limitations to the diagnostic capability of CT remain. Although

the addition of CT-guided biopsy has demonstrated the potential of CT imaging for pre-autopsy histopathological diagnosis in small studies, additional investigations are needed to validate its diagnostic role in more cases with various causes of death.[10-12] However, both autopsy and PMCT/PMCTA are imperfect; autopsy and CT imaging may occasionally be unable to identify all injuries related to the cause of death. Notably, additional perimortem therapeutic interventions can interfere with the detection of original complications during CT examination and autopsy dissection. In this regard, CT imaging and autopsy should be performed in a complementary manner to establish accurately the cause of death in fatal cases with medicolegal components.

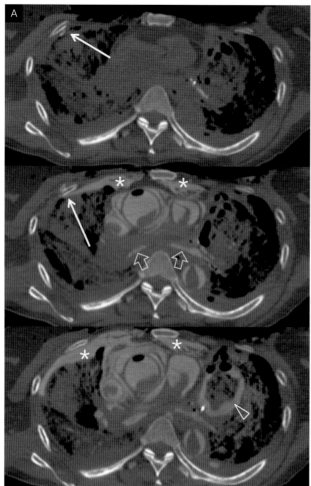
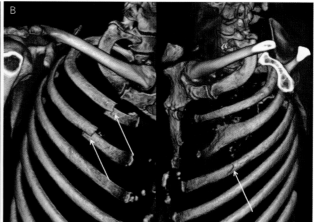

Figure 6. Massive hemoptysis that occurred 1 week after left upper lobectomy.

(A) Compared with noncontrast-enhanced image (upper), postmortem CT angiography shows systemic arterial bleeding (arrow) into the bronchial lumens (arrows) after arterial injection of a contrast agent (middle) and venous bleeding into the lung parenchyma (arrowhead) after subsequent venous injection (low). Note the presence of a fracture (long arrows) at the anterolateral angle of the rib and contrast leakage into the anterior chest wall (*) on axial image. (B) Three-dimensional volume-rendered coronal (left) and oblique sagittal (right) images show multiple rib fractures associated with cardiopulmonary resuscitation (long arrows).

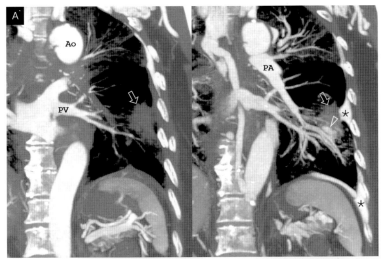

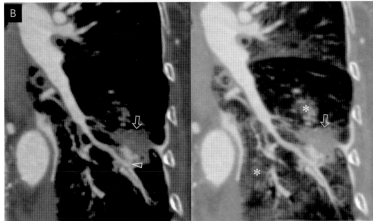

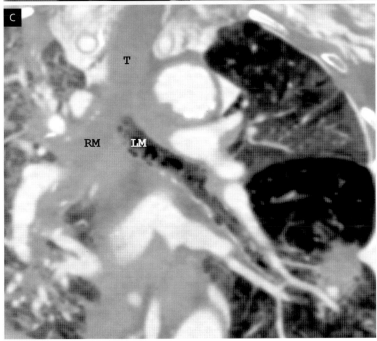

Figure 7. Fatal hemorrhage after percutaneous needle biopsy of a lung nodule.

Oblique coronal images were reconstructed using MIP (A) and MPR (B, C) techniques. An 84-year-old female died of massive hemoptysis after transthoracic needle biopsy of a lung nodule.

(A) After retrograde contrast injection into the femoral artery, a maximum intensity projection image shows the contrast filled left atrium and pulmonary veins (left). After antegrade injection into the femoral vein, pulmonary arteries were opacified and contrast leakage (arrowhead) into the nodule (arrow) was demonstrated (right), indicating pulmonary arterial injury as the source of fatal hemorrhage. (B) Curved MPR image pinpoints the site of the vascular injury (arrowhead) and contrast leakage into the lung nodule (arrows) and surrounding parenchymal hemorrhage (* in right). (C) MPR image shows the luminal occlusion of trachea and right mainstem bronchus filled with densities ranging 20-50HU, suggestive of blood clot.

MPR: multiplanar reformation, MIP: maximum intensity projection

PV: pulmonary vein, Ao: Aorta, PA: pulmonary artery, T: trachea, LM: left mainstem bronchus, RM: right mainstem bronchus.

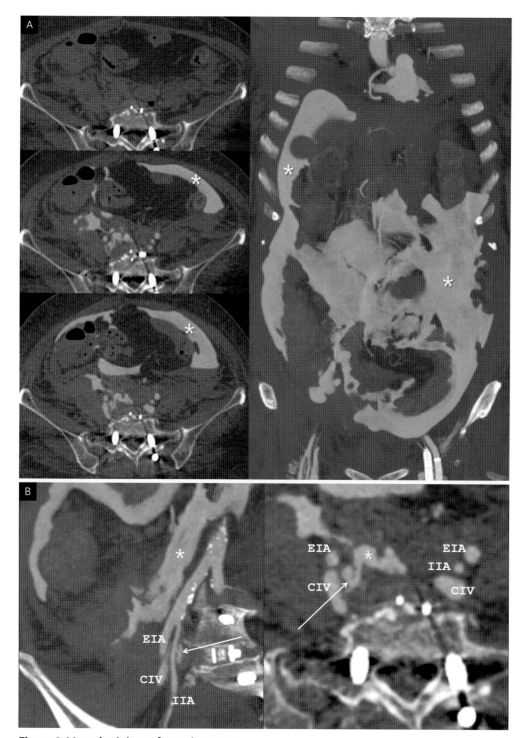

Figure 8. Vascular injury after spine surgery.

(A) Axial images (left row) of nonenhanced postmortem CT (upper) and CT angiography with arterial (middle) and subsequent venous injection (lower) show contrast leakage into the abdominal cavity (*) after arterial injection of contrast agent (middle), suggesting arterial bleeding. Coronal image (right) reconstructed with maximum intensity projection shows extensive contrast leakage into the abdominal cavity. (B) Oblique coronal (left) and axial (right) images show focal rupture of the internal iliac artery (arrow) and contrast leakage (*). EIA: external iliac artery, IIA: internal iliac artery, CIV: common iliac vein

Summary

In cases of unexpected death after medical intervention, postmortem CT imaging can provide pre-autopsy screening for potential injuries and guide careful exposure of the lesion during autopsy to add visual and histological analysis without destroying evidence.

References

1 Heinemann A, Vogel H, Heller M, Tzikas A, Püschel K. Investigation of medical intervention with fatal outcome: the impact of post-mortem CT and CT angiography. La Radiologia medica. 2015; 120(9):835-45. doi: 10.1007/s11547-015-0574-5.

2 Zerlauth JB, Doenz F, Dominguez A, Palmiere C, Uské A, Meuli R, et al. Surgical interventions with fatal outcome: utility of multiphase postmortem CT angiography. Forensic science international. 2013; 225(1-3):32-41. doi: 10.1016/j.forsciint.2012.05.013.

3 Wichmann D, Obbelode F, Vogel H, Hoepker WW, Nierhaus A, Braune S, et al. Virtual autopsy as an alternative to traditional medical autopsy in the intensive care unit: a prospective cohort study. Annals of internal medicine. 2012;156(2):123-30. doi: 10.7326/0003-4819-156-2-201201170-00008.

4 Wichmann D, Heinemann A, Weinberg C, Vogel H, Hoepker WW, Grabherr S, et al. Virtual autopsy with multiphase postmortem computed tomographic angiography versus traditional medical autopsy to investigate unexpected deaths of hospitalized patients: a cohort study. Annals of internal medicine. 2014;160(8):534-41. doi: 10.7326/m13-2211.

5 Grabherr S, Egger C, Vilarino R, Campana L, Jotterand M, Dedouit F. Modern post-mortem imaging: an update on recent developments. Forensic sciences research. 2017;2(2):52-64. doi: 10.1080/20961790.2017.1330738.

6 Vogel B, Heinemann A, Tzikas A, Poodendaen C, Gulbins H, Reichenspurner H, et al. Post-mortem computed tomography (PMCT) and PMCT-angiography after cardiac surgery. Possibilities and limits. Archiwum medycyny sadowej i kryminologii. 2013;63(3): 155-71. doi: 10.5114/amsik.2013.46124.

7 Grabherr S, Grimm J, Dominguez A, Vanhaebost J, Mangin P. Advances in post-mortem CT-angiography. The British journal of radiology. 2014;87(1036):20130488. doi: 10.1259/bjr.20130488.

8 Ross SG, Bolliger SA, Ampanozi G, Oesterhelweg L, Thali MJ, Flach PM. Postmortem CT angiography: capabilities and limitations in traumatic and natural causes of death. Radiographics: a review publication of the Radiological Society of North America, Inc. 2014; 34(3):830-46. doi: 10.1148/rg.343115169.

9 Bruguier C, Mosimann PJ, Vaucher P, Uské A, Doenz F, Jackowski C, et al. Multi-phase postmortem CT angiography: recognizing technique-related artefacts and pitfalls. International journal of legal medicine. 2013;127(3):639-52. doi: 10.1007/s00414-013-0840-9.

10 Lee H, Lee S, Cha JG, Baek T, Yang KM. Postmortem Computed Tomography and Computed Tomography Angiography: Cardiothoracic Imaging Applications in Forensic Medicine. Journal of thoracic imaging. 2019;34(5):286-98. doi: 10.1097/rti.0000000000000398.

11 Ross SG, Thali MJ, Bolliger S, Germerott T, Ruder TD, Flach PM. Sudden death after chest pain: feasibility of virtual autopsy with postmortem CT angiography and biopsy. Radiology. 2012;264(1): 250-9. doi: 10.1148/radiol.12092415.

12 Bolliger SA, Filograna L, Spendlove D, Thali MJ, Dirnhofer S, Ross S. Postmortem imaging-guided biopsy as an adjuvant to minimally invasive autopsy with CT and postmortem angiography: a feasibility study. AJR American journal of roentgenology. 2010;195(5):1051-6. doi: 10.2214/ajr.10.4600.

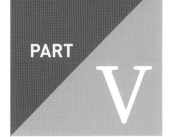

PART

V

Artifacts frequently found on postmortem CT and CTA

He who would distinguish between true and
false must have an adequate idea of true and false.
– Baruch Spinoza, 1632–1677

Chapter 11

Perimortem intervention and CTA-specific artifacts

Since the adoption of CT and CT angiographic techniques in death investigations, various CT imaging findings that could mimic true pathologies have been described. These artifacts are mostly related to perimortem medical interventions (e.g., cardiopulmonary resuscitation, CPR) or postmortem body changes that begin immediately after death but vary among personal and environmental situations. Therefore, knowledge of the potential sources of artifacts and their imaging findings is important for adequate interpretation of postmortem CT images, thus avoiding misidentification as true pathologies.[1]

11.1. Perimortem medical intervention

Perimortem CPR can produce many iatrogenic artifacts, including fractures of the ribs and sternum, injuries of the heart and lungs, and air collection in heart chambers and vessels on CT imaging. These findings should not be mistaken for primary traumatic lesions that led to CPR. Rib fractures are commonly associated with chest wall injuries. In cases of blunt chest trauma, most rib fractures are found at the fourth to seventh ribs in the lateral and posterolateral aspects on both sides although depending on the site of impact.[2] In contrast, CPR-related rib fractures are usually detected in the anterolateral angles of the second to sixth ribs in a bilaterally symmetrical manner. Sternal fractures usually occur at the level of the third to fifth sternocostal junctions, which is the body location of corresponding rib fractures.[3] Major cardiac injuries may occur in relation to rib and sternal fractures, following standard CPR (Figs. 1 and 2).

Among the cardiac chambers, the right ventricle is reportedly most susceptible to rupture due to increased pressure, followed by the right atrium. Although the exact frequency is unknown, CPR-related cardiac injuries are not uncommon in CPR non-survivors in our daily practice.

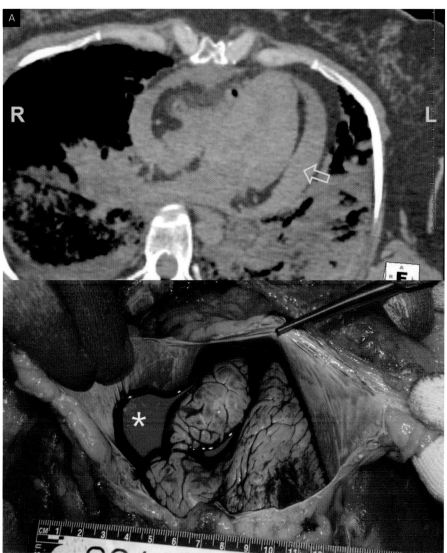

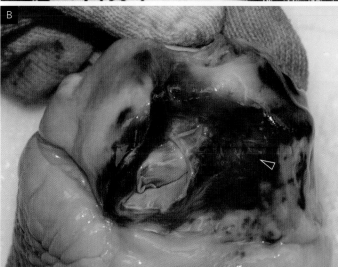

Figure 1. Cardiopulmonary resuscitation (CPR)-related cardiac injury

(A) Axial image of postmortem CT shows pericardial hemorrhage (arrow) without the "hyperdense armored heart" sign (hyperdense ring from coagulation on a beating epicardial surface), indicative of heartbeat cessation during bleeding into the pericardial cavity in this case. Autopsy photograph confirms non-coagulated blood in the pericardial cavity (*). (B) Focal rupture of the right atrium (arrowhead) was identified during autopsy. In our experience, CPR-related heart injuries (e.g., right atrial or ventricular rupture) are not uncommon in non-survivors of CPR.

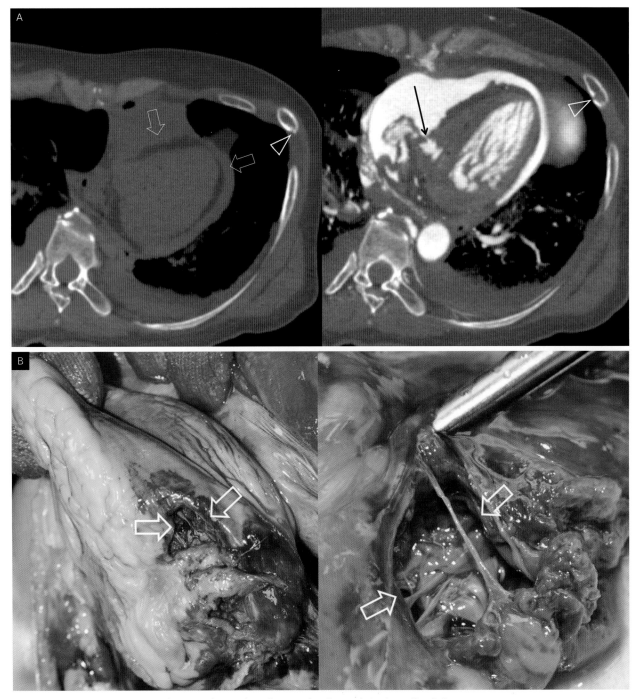

Figure 2. Postmortem CT and CT angiography of resuscitation-related cardiac injury.
(A) Axial image of postmortem CT (left) shows hemopericardium without the hyperdense ring (arrows) caused by coagulation. After intravascular contrast injection, focal rupture (long black arrow) of the right atrial wall and contrast leakage into the pericardium are visible. Note the presence of rib fracture (arrowhead) at the anterolateral angle.
(B) Photographs of the autopsy specimen show focal rupture of the right atrium (arrows).

11.2. Artifacts related to PMCTA and angiography techniques

11.2.1. Postmortem clots

By definition, a blood clot is a clump of coagulated blood that seals an injured blood vessel as the final step of normal hemostasis.[4, 5] Thrombus refers to a blood clot formed within a blood vessel by one of several distinct causes, including Virchow's triad. When a thrombus dislodges and travels to another location, it is regarded as an embolus and increases the risk of vascular obstruction.[6] A postmortem clot refers to a simple aggregation of blood components within the vascular system after death, which comprises the remnants of blood cells and fibrin that clump in a random manner. Postmortem clots are gelatinous, rubbery, and easily removed because they are not attached to the vessel wall.[5, 7] In contrast, thrombi are harder but fragile and adhere to the vessel wall. Microscopically, thrombi have a laminated appearance (i.e., lines of Zahn) of alternating dark layers of red blood cells and light layers of platelets mixed with fibrin[5], characteristic of antemortem thrombosis at the point of rapid blood flow.[8]

The cessation of blood flow after death induces clotting processes that form postmortem clots, because fibrinogen and platelets remain viable and functional for a period of time after death.[7, 9] Although postmortem clotting occurs predominantly within cardiac chambers and great vessels (e.g., pulmonary arteries, right heart, and aorta).[1, 10], widespread clotting can be found in cases with a prolonged period of pain and suffering (agony).[7, 11] Notably, minimal clotting occurs in cases with a short time to death, reportedly due to high plasma levels of catecholamine and plasminogen activators that induce thrombolysis.[7, 12]

Postmortem clots can also be observed during PMCTA as low-density filling defects within the vascular system. Therefore, postmortem clotting should be carefully assessed to avoid misinterpretation as antemortem thrombus **(Fig. 3)**.

Although contrast defects from the pulmonary trunk to the main pulmonary arteries are reportedly more likely to represent a thromboembolus than a postmortem clot, any vascular filling defect can be caused by a thromboembolus or postmortem clot, which generally occur in these locations.[1, 10] Accordingly, the etiology of intravascular filling defects can only be validated with histological examination, although PMCT can be used to guide percutaneous biopsy to obtain the tissue sample and provide additional histopathological information regarding these filling defects.[12] Furthermore, in cases where very few clots or extensive clots in the heart and vessels are found during PMCTA, the degree of postmortem clotting in images can be used as a clue to support or rule out sudden death if the use of anticoagulants can be excluded.[7]

11.2.2. Artifacts related to the use of contrast agents

Postmortem vascular changes include the cessation of circulation, increased permeability of the vascular walls, and the presence of collapsed vessels that are empty or partially filled with postmortem clots and gas. Therefore, a considerable amount of contrast is needed to fill and expand the vascular

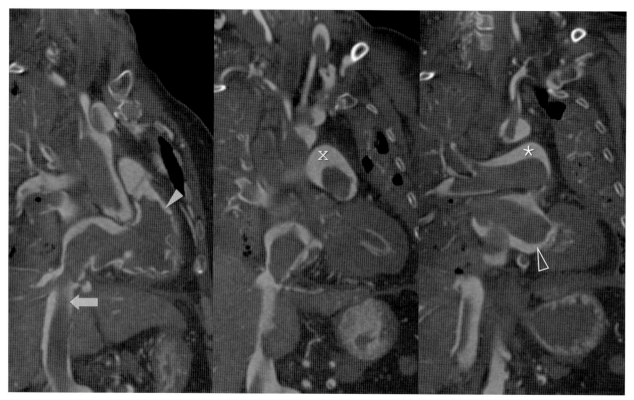

Figure 3. Postmortem clots.
Oblique coronal images (from anterior to posterior direction) of postmortem CT angiography show extensive mass-like low-density filling defects molded into the luminal shape of the pulmonary trunk (x), right pulmonary artery (*), left atrium (arrowhead), inferior vena cava (white arrow), and right ventricle (white-filled arrowhead).

system to achieve its original dimension. Currently, the most popular contrast agents for PMCTA are iodinated water-soluble agents and iodized oil. These are mixed with hydrophilic polyethylene glycol (PEG) and paraffin oil, respectively, for use as contrast dissolvers, perfusates, and volume expanders.[13]

Contrast leakage at the site of autolysis

Early contrast leakage may be observed at sites of early autolysis, especially in cases where fat-soluble contrast agents were injected. Autolysis of the pancreas and stomach begins immediately after death

and results in vessel wall damage due to the digestive action of their own enzymes. Although oily contrast mixture has the advantage of longer retention in undamaged vessels, compared with water-soluble mixtures, it can rapidly extravasate through the damaged vascular wall. Thus, the correct diagnosis of true injuries in these areas may be difficult. However, in cases where water-soluble contrast mixture is used, large PEG molecules in the mixture increase the viscosity of the contrast solution, reducing extravasation through the damaged vessel wall **(Fig.4)**.[1, 13]

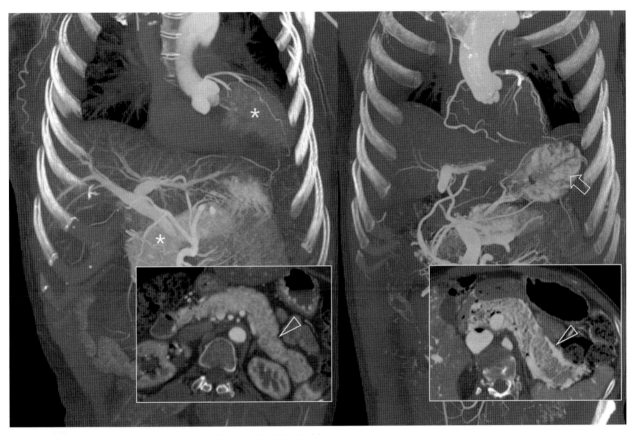

Figure 4. Characteristics of water-soluble and lipid-soluble agents.
Postmortem CT angiography performed after arterial injection of water-soluble (left) and lipid-soluble (right) contrast agents. Diffuse organ parenchymal enhancement (* and arrowhead in left) is prominent when a water-soluble agent is used because of extravascular diffusion, but contrast leakage from the organs (i.e., where early autolysis begins immediately after death) through damaged vessel walls is remarkable when lipid-soluble agents are used (arrowhead in right).

Extravascular contrast diffusion

After the injection of a water-soluble mixture, prominent parenchymal enhancement is found in solid organs (e.g., brain, heart, liver, and kidneys); this is attributable to the extravascular diffusion of small water-soluble iodized molecules, while larger PEG molecules remain in the vessels (**Fig. 4**). Because the rapid vascular diffusion leads to a rapid reduction in the degree of vascular enhancement, the recommended delay between injection and scanning is ≤ 20 min when using a water-soluble mixture.[10]

Furthermore, contrast mixing with blood may interfere with efforts to quantify the volume of hemorrhagic blood.[1, 14]

Blood clumping

The hygroscopic nature of hyperosmolar water-soluble contrast mixtures induces widespread blood clumping in the vascular system, specifically by attracting water from the surrounding environment, which may interfere with the diagnosis of thrombus during autopsy dissection.[14]

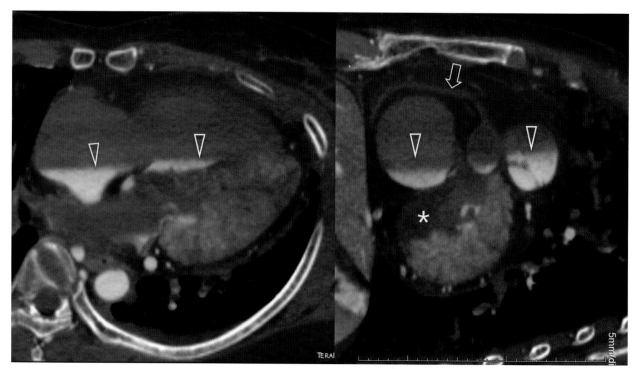

Figure 5. Postmortem CT angiography performed using a water-soluble contrast agent.
Axial (left) and oblique coronal (right) CT images show that the contrast agent is collected in the dependent position of cardiac chambers (arrowheads) due to its higher specific gravity, compared with blood. Therefore, the right coronary artery (arrow) may be incompletely filled with contrast agent, resulting in a myocardial contrast defect (*) in the lower wall of the left ventricle if the body is not moved to the prone position before scanning.

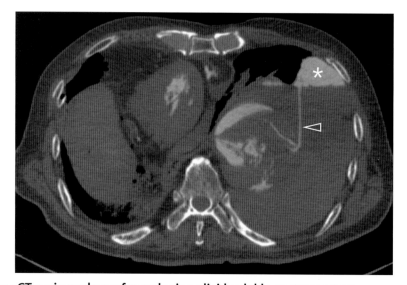

Figure 6. Postmortem CT angiography performed using a lipid-soluble contrast agent.
Axial CT image shows direct leakage (arrowhead) of the contrast medium from a ruptured aneurysm into the pleural cavity. Because the contrast agent is lighter than the blood collected in the pleural cavity, it accumulates in a non-dependent location in the pleural cavity (*).

Specific gravities of contrast media

Similar to clinical contrast agents, hydrophilic contrast mixtures are based on water-soluble iodinated molecules that are used for clinical radiology and have higher specific gravity, compared with blood.[1]When CT acquisition is performed without movement of the body to a prone position, certain body locations may not be completely filled with contrast medium. A notable example is the right coronary artery, which is least dependent in the supine position **(Fig. 5)**.[10]

In contrast, when lipid-soluble contrast is injected, it is lighter than blood, thus leading to contrast leakage into a non-dependent position **(Fig. 6)**.

11.3. Summary

Accurate interpretation of postmortem images requires knowledge and understanding of a variety of artifacts related to perimortem resuscitation and PMCTA techniques, as well as postmortem tissue changes, which are often encountered during image analyses and may mimic true pathologies. Therefore, familiarity with these artifacts is essential to prevent misinterpretation and to ensure the greatest benefits from PMCT and PMCTA techniques during death investigations.

References

1   Lee H, Lee S, Cha JG, Baek T, Yang KM. Postmortem Computed Tomography and Computed Tomography Angiography: Cardiothoracic Imaging Applications in Forensic Medicine. Journal of thoracic imaging. 2019;34(5):286-98. doi: 10.1097/rti.0000000000000398.

2   Liebsch C, Seiffert T, Vlcek M, Beer M, Huber-Lang M, Wilke HJ. Patterns of serial rib fractures after blunt chest trauma: An analysis of 380 cases. PloS one. 2019;14(12):e0224105. doi: 10.1371/journal.pone.0224105.

3   Deliliga A, Chatzinikolaou F, Koutsoukis D, Chrysovergis I, Voultsos P. Cardiopulmonary resuscitation (CPR) complications encountered in forensic autopsy cases. BMC emergency medicine. 2019; 19(1):23. doi: 10.1186/s12873-019-0234-5.

4   Quinn JG, Tansey EA, Johnson CD, Roe SM, Montgomery LE. Blood: tests used to assess the physiological and immunological properties of blood. Advances in physiology education. 2016;40(2):165-75. doi: 10.1152/advan.00079.2015.

5   Thrombosis. In: Bang NU, Beller FK, Deutsch E, Mammen EF, editors. Thrombosis and Bleeding Disorders. Academic Press; 1971. p. 488-534.

6   Ashorobi D, Ameer M, Fernandez R. Thrombosis..[Updated 2020 Oct 3] In: StatPearls.[Internet] Treasure Island (FL): StatPearls Publishing. 2020-Jan-. https://www.ncbi.nlm.nih.gov/books/NBK538430/.

7   Jackowski C, Thali M, Aghayev E, Yen K, Sonnenschein M, Zwygart K, et al. Postmortem imaging of blood and its characteristics using MSCT and MRI. International journal of legal medicine. 2006; 120(4):233-40. doi: 10.1007/s00414-005-0023-4.

8   Lee R, Adlam D, Clelland CA, Channon KM. Lines of Zahn in coronary artery thrombus. European heart journal. 2012;33(9):1039. doi: 10.1093/eurheartj/ehs028.

9   Thomsen H, Krisch B. The postmortem activation status of platelets. International journal of legal medicine. 1994;107(3):111-7. doi: 10.1007/bf01225596.

10 Ross SG, Bolliger SA, Ampanozi G, Oesterhelweg L, Thali MJ, Flach PM. Postmortem CT angiography: capabilities and limitations in traumatic and natural causes of death. Radiographics : a review publication of the Radiological Society of North America, Inc. 2014; 34(3):830-46. doi: 10.1148/rg.343115169.

11 Bruguier C, Mosimann PJ, Vaucher P, Uské A, Doenz F, Jackowski C, et al. Multi-phase postmortem CT angiography: recognizing technique-related artefacts and pitfalls. International journal of legal medicine. 2013;127(3):639-52. doi: 10.1007/s00414-013-0840-9.

12 Ross SG, Thali MJ, Bolliger S, Germerott T, Ruder TD, Flach PM. Sudden death after chest pain: feasibility of virtual autopsy with postmortem CT angiography and biopsy. Radiology. 2012;264(1):250-9. doi: 10.1148/radiol.12092415.

13 Ross S, Spendlove D, Bolliger S, Christe A, Oesterhelweg L, Grabherr S, et al. Postmortem whole-body CT angiography: evaluation of two contrast media solutions. AJR American journal of roentgenology. 2008;190(5):1380-9. doi: 10.2214/ajr.07.3082.

14 Grabherr S, Grimm J, Baumann P, Mangin P. Application of contrast media in post-mortem imaging (CT and MRI). La Radiologia medica. 2015;120(9):824-34. doi: 10.1007/s11547-015-0532-2.

Chapter 12

Decomposition

In contrast to clinical CT imaging, multiple death-related artifacts (e.g., postmortem changes and decomposition) are always found on postmortem CT (PMCT). These pathological alterations begin immediately after death and thus have the potential to mask underlying pathologies or to be misinterpreted as true lesions, complicating diagnostics during PMCT and during traditional autopsy. Therefore, it is essential to have knowledge of these "normal" postmortem processes in terms of their types, times of onset, and distributions. This knowledge can prevent the misdiagnosis of those findings as abnormal, and can prevent the misinterpretation of true pathologies as natural postmortem processes. Although the identification and examination of decomposed bodies are currently challenging, PMCT has can provide additional diagnostic information beyond visual assessment for the forensic investigation of severely decomposed cases.

Although postmortem changes comprise livor mortis (i.e., postmortem hypostasis or hemoconcen-

tration), rigor mortis (i.e., postmortem rigidity), and algor mortis (i.e., postmortem change in body temperature to match the environmental temperature), livor mortis is the only postmortem change that can be identified on CT. It is the pooling of stagnant blood, particularly erythrocytes, in the body due to gravity when blood circulation stops after heartbeat cessation.[1, 2] This gravity-dependent distribution and extent of hemoconcentration depends on the body position after death and becomes visible at 20 min to 2 h after death, reaching its maximum at 12 h before becoming fixed at the initial position.[3, 4]

Decomposition refers to the breakdown of dead organic tissue into simpler organic or inorganic materials (e.g., water, gas, and mineral salts). It is a multifactorial process that is caused by cellular autolysis and putrefaction (bacterial fermentation), which also begins at the moment of death.[1] Cellular autolysis is the temperature-dependent breakdown of cells through the actions of their own internal proteolytic enzymes. Autolysis is accelerated by

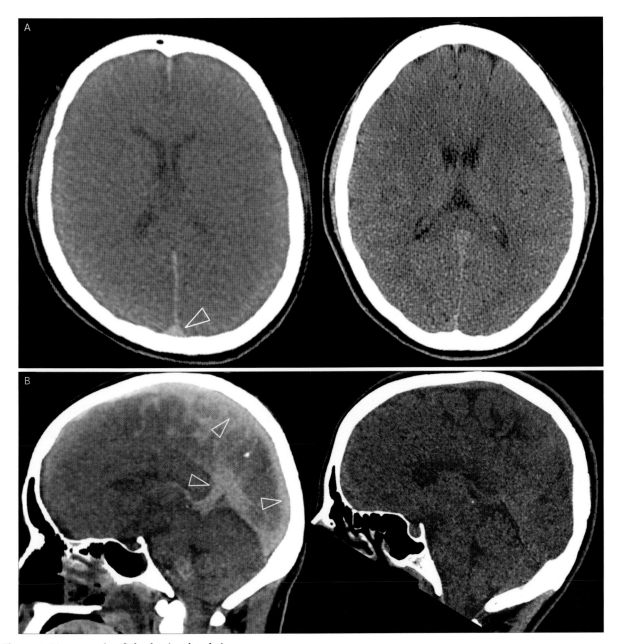

Figure 1. Hypostasis of the brain: dural sinus.

Axial (left in A) and sagittal (left in B) images show hyperdense dural sinus (arrowheads) due to dependent hemoconcentration. For comparison, note the differences in images compared with an antemortem case (right image in A and B).

higher temperature and humidity, but slowed by low temperature and completely stops in freezing conditions.[3] In contrast to the body surface, internal organ autolysis processes occur at different rates. Pancreatic and adrenal autolysis processes begin almost immediately after death. The brain is susceptible to autolysis and liquefies within 1 week after death. In contrast, the myocardium, vessels, uterus, and prostate are comparatively less vulnerable to autolysis and remain recognizable for an extended duration.[1, 2] Putrefaction refers to a complex chemical process caused by microorganisms, which leads to tissue breakdown and gas accumulation within the body. Normal gastrointestinal flora and pathogenic bacte-

ria within the body induce putrefaction throughout the body. The rate of putrefaction varies among tissues and is dependent on numerous interrelated factors. Internal factors influencing putrefaction include age at death, cause of death, overall body condition (size and weight), and external body injuries. External factors that may affect the rate of putrefaction include environmental temperature, humidity, clothing, soil or surface on which the dead body is located, burial factors, and predation by animals or insects.[5]

On PMCT, gravity-dependent hemoconcentration results in increased attenuation in affected vessels, tissues, and organs. This feature is observed in

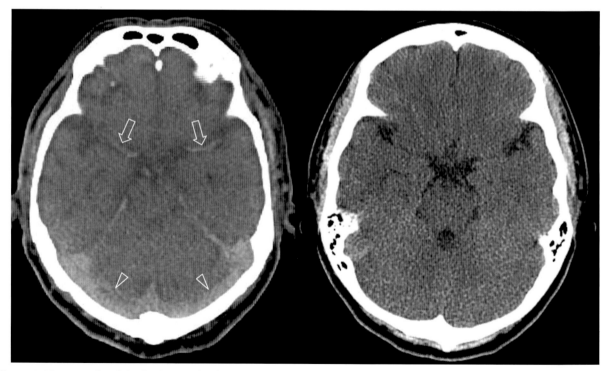

Figure 2. Hypostasis of the brain: cerebral arteries.
Axial image (left) of postmortem CT shows hyperdense middle cerebral arteries (arrows) due to hemoconcentration. Compare with an image from an antemortem case (right), and note the high densities of dural sinuses (arrowheads) due to dependent hemoconcentration.

half of the cases examined within 2 h after death (**Figs. 1-3**).[6]

The earliest sign of decomposition is brain autolysis (**Fig. 4**), regardless of body storage in a cooling chamber (24-48 h).

The pancreas and adrenal glands are internal organs that undergo early autolysis, although they remain normal on PMCT until putrefactive gas is identified.[1] Gastromalacia is a type of early postmortem autolysis that can result in gastric perforation (e.g., in the posterior wall of the gastric fundus) caused by endogenous gastric enzymes, which leads

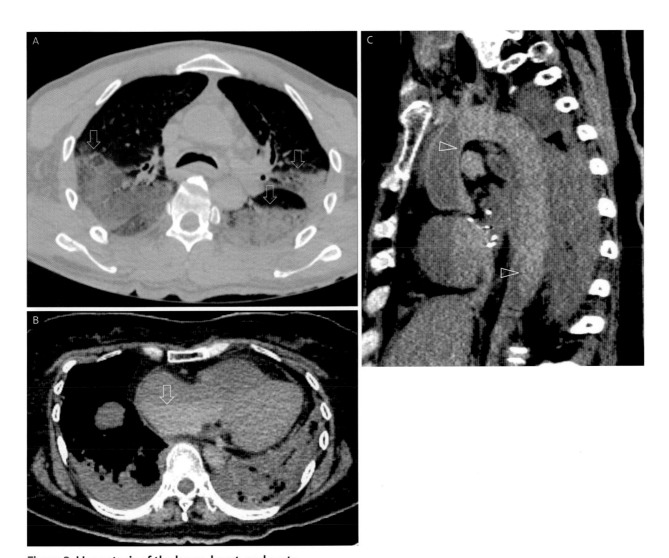

Figure 3. Hypostasis of the lungs, heart, and aorta.
(A) Postmortem axial CT image shows a gradual increase in the density of lung parenchyma from the non-dependent position to the dependent position in lung window settings. Note the presence of nearly horizontal borders (arrows) of increased attenuations. (B, C) Postmortem axial (B) and sagittal (C) CT images show layered high density in the right atrium (arrow) and aorta with horizontal borders (arrowheads) of increased attenuations.

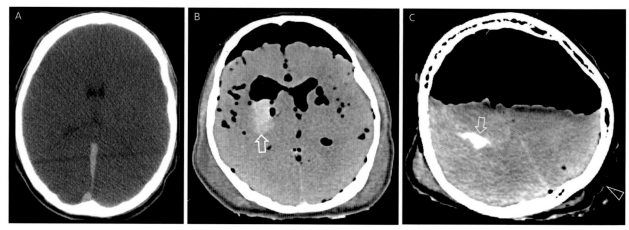

Figure 4. Classification of decomposition in the brain.
Axial images of postmortem CT show (A) the effacement of sulci and complete loss of gray-white matter differentiation during early decomposition; (B) settling of the brain in dependent positions and putrefactive gas filling in non-dependent positions in the cranial cavity, vasculature, and soft tissue of the scalp (not shown in this image) during moderate decomposition; and finally, (C) liquefaction of the brain with an air-fluid level, putrefactive gas filling in the cranial cavity and soft tissue, and the scalp having peeled away from the calvarium (arrowhead) during advanced decomposition. Note the presence of antemortem hemorrhage in the brain parenchyma (arrows in B and C).

to pneumoperitoneum or pneumothorax and thus mimics antemortem injury.[7] This entity is frequently encountered by forensic pathologists, but is unfamiliar to clinical radiologists.

Putrefaction is indirectly revealed by its gas formation on CT images. This minimally invasive tool shows gaseous accumulation and distension of the putrefied tissue and organs within 5–84 h after death.[8] Although occasionally difficult because the rate of putrefaction is highly variable and may be modified by the body's location, analysis of the pattern of gas distribution in a corpse may enable distinction between putrefactive gas and potentially lethal vascular air embolism. Intestinal wall and mesenteric and portal venous systems are the first sites of putrefactive gas on PMCT, followed by right heart chambers

(Figs. 5-9).[8]

However, the rate of decomposition is highly variable; it is frequently modified by the location of the body and the surrounding environment (Figs. 9 and 10).

PMCT is also useful in identifying complex fractures of bony structures and screening for foreign materials in putrefied bodies by means of whole-body scanning. Moreover, with respect to advanced stages of decomposition, PMCT is valuable for identification of the body and provides additional benefits in terms of depicting relevant findings and diagnosing some pathological findings in a more precise manner (e.g., intracranial hemorrhage, hemopericardium, and hemothorax), either in superficial or deep locations (Figs. 11-14).

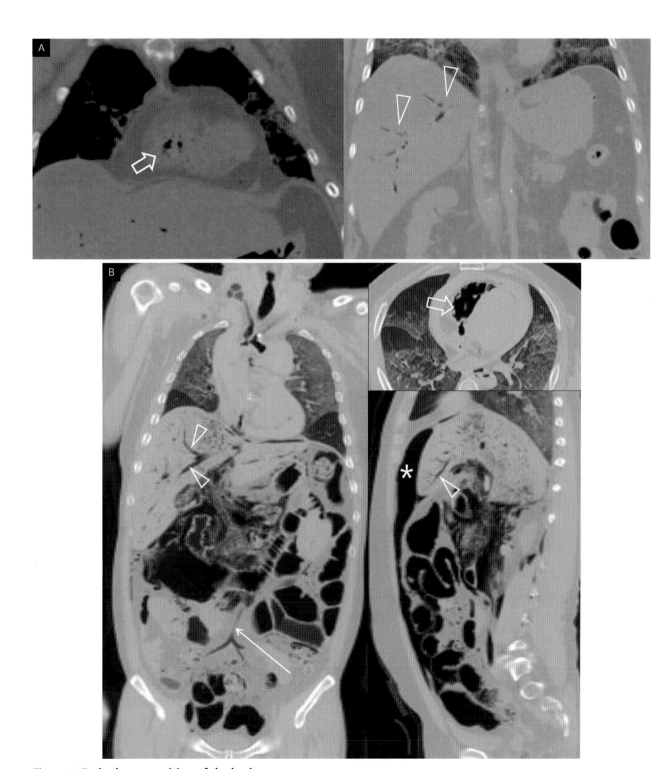

Figure 5. Early decomposition of the body.
(A) Coronal images of chest (left) and upper abdomen (right). (B) Coronal image of trunk (left), axial image of heart (right upper), and sagittal image (right lower) of abdomen. In these two cases, postmortem CT shows gas in the portal vein within the liver (arrowheads in A and B), right heart (arrows in a and b), mesenteric vessels (long arrow in B), and peritoneal cavity (* in B), which comprise the first sites where putrefactive gas appears.

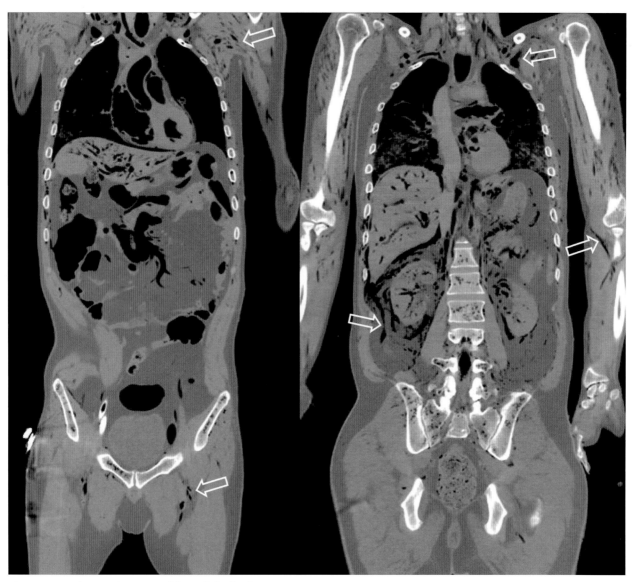

Figure 6. Moderate decomposition of the body.
Coronal CT images of the trunk from anterior (left) to posterior (right) show multifocal gas collection in various tissue planes (arrows), as well as in the cardiac chambers and portal veins within the liver.

In clinical radiology, CT is the first-line imaging modality used to evaluate patients with suspected ICH, mostly based on density differences between a hematoma and the brain parenchyma. The density of intracranial hemorrhage changes over time, reflecting clot formation, retraction, and lysis. Therefore, density changes are used to estimate the age of hemorrhagic blood, ranging from hyperacute to chronic stages. Initially, freshly extravasated blood shows a mixed attenuation ranging from 40 to 60 HU immediately after bleeding. Then, CT attenuation of the hematoma increases to 80-100 HU with a meshwork formation of fibrin and globin, followed by clot maturation and retraction. Within a few weeks after initial bleeding, the hematoma attenuation value decreases daily, due to the chemical decomposition of globin molecules and subsequent phagocytosis by macrophages, eventually leading to complete resolu-

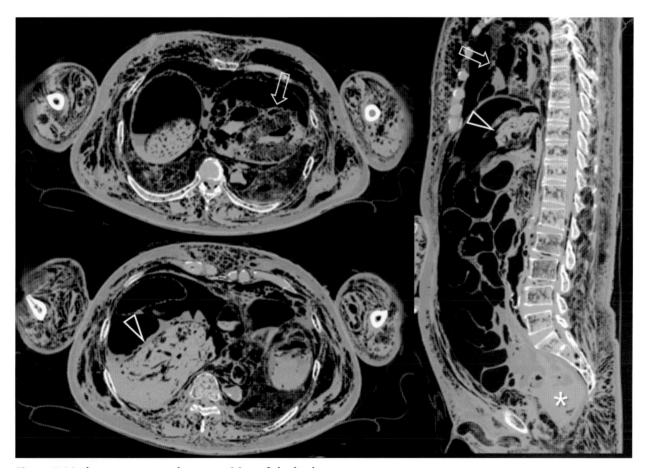

Figure 7. Moderate to severe decomposition of the body.
Axial images at the level of the heart (left upper) and liver (left lower) show extensive putrefactive gas throughout the vasculature, all tissue planes, and all body cavities. These images also depict the partial collapse of organs such as the heart (arrows) and liver (arrowheads). Note the presence of gas in pericardial, pleural, and peritoneal cavities, as well as in the cardiac chambers, retroperitoneal space, and subcutaneous tissue; small fluid collection (*) is evident in the pelvic cavity.

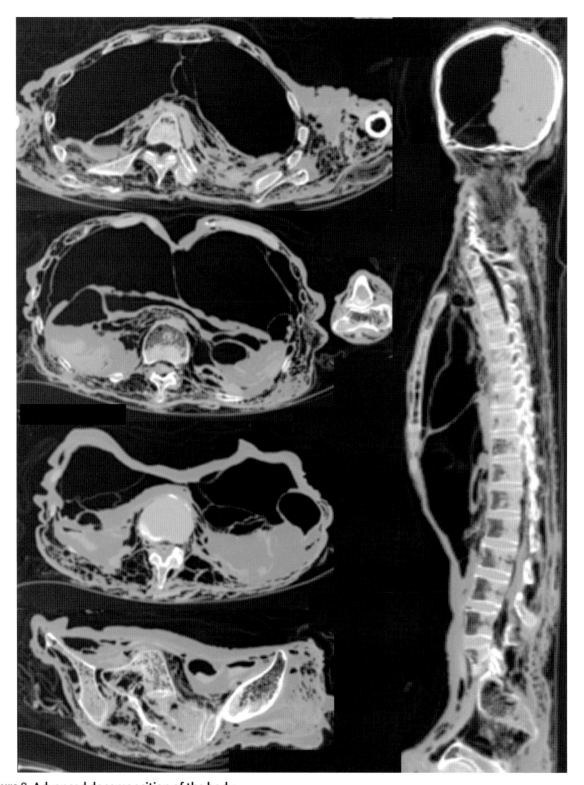

Figure 8. Advanced decomposition of the body.
Axial (left) images from the chest to pelvis and sagittal (right) image of the head and trunk show collapse of the brain, lungs, liver, and other abdominopelvic organs; the images also show gas throughout all tissue planes.

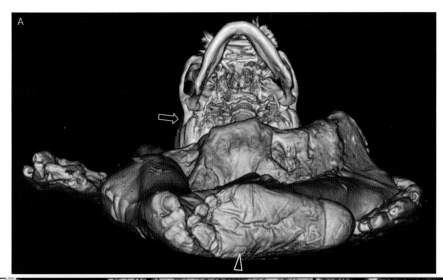

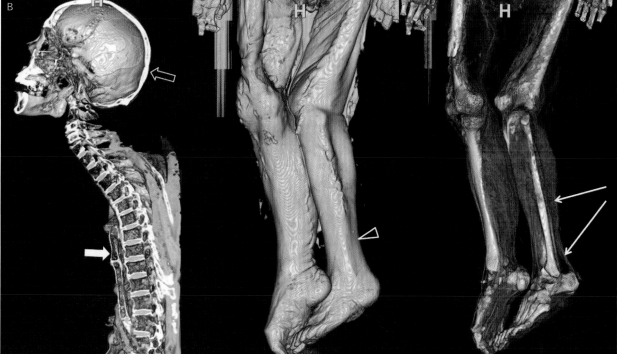

Figure 9. Asymmetrical decomposition of the body.
(A) 3D VR image viewed from below shows advanced decomposition of the head exposing the skull (arrow), but demonstrates preservation of skin and soft tissue within the extremities (arrowhead). (B) Lateral (left) and anterolateral views (middle and right) of 3D VR images show advanced decomposition of the head (arrow) and trunk (white arrow) with multi-organ collapse; the views also demonstrate mild to moderate decomposition of the lower extremities with well-preserved muscles and tendons (long arrows) under the skin (arrowheads). The decomposition rate depends mainly on three groups of factors: the physical environment (i.e., temperature, humidity, burial depth, and soil properties), the dead body itself (i.e., cause of death, size and weight of the body, and clothing), and the nature of microorganisms within and surrounding the body. Furthermore, locally accelerated or delayed decomposition occurs when part of the body is placed or covered in a manner that creates a local environment promoting or inhibiting decomposition, thereby causing asymmetrical decomposition. 3D VR: Three-dimensional volume-rendered

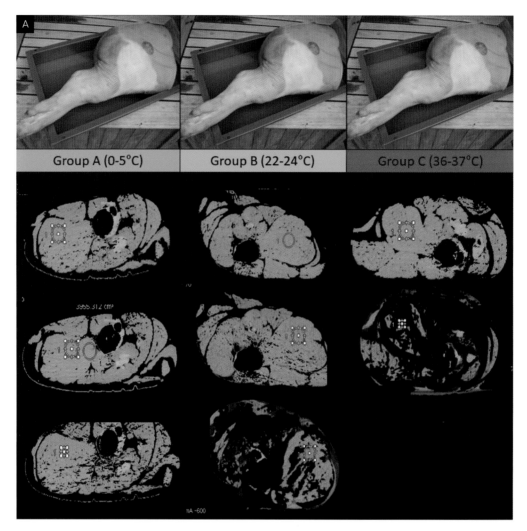

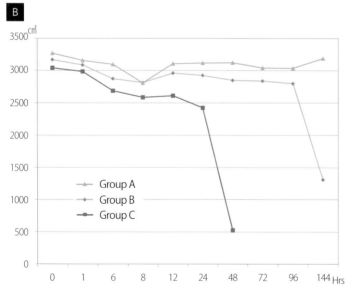

Figure 10. Effect of temperature on decomposition rate.

(A) Three pork hind legs were obtained within 12 h after slaughter. These legs were stored at different temperatures: low (0-5°C), moderate (i.e., room temperature; 22-24°C), and high (36-37°C). Serial CT acquisition was performed and data were analyzed to calculate muscle mass. Note the reduction of soft tissue density and the enhancement of air density, corresponding to muscle and decomposition gases in the legs, respectively.
(B) A graph based on CT data shows a rapid reduction in muscle volume within 2 days at high temperature, due to decomposition. In contrast, muscle volume does not change noticeably over the course of 1 week at cold temperature. On the sixth day at room temperature, muscle mass began to visibly decrease (unpublished data).

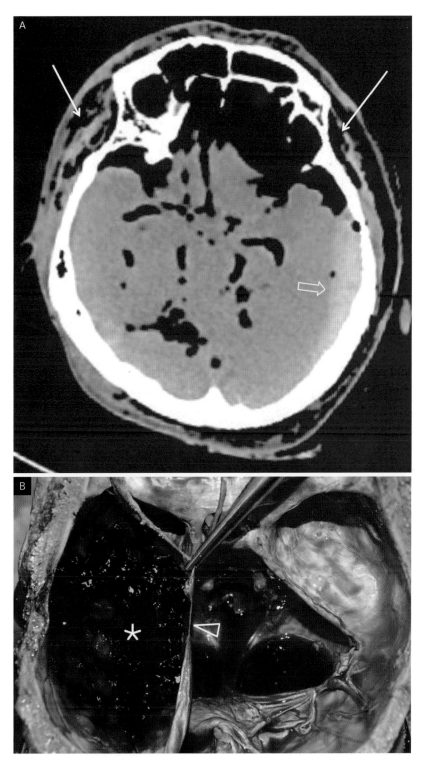

Figure 11. Epidural hematoma in a decomposed case.
(A) Axial image of postmortem CT shows epidural hematoma (arrow) in the left temporal area. Note the presence of scalp (long arrows) that has peeled away from the calvarium due to advanced decomposition. (B) Autopsy specimen depicts dura mater (arrowhead) and epidural hematoma (*).

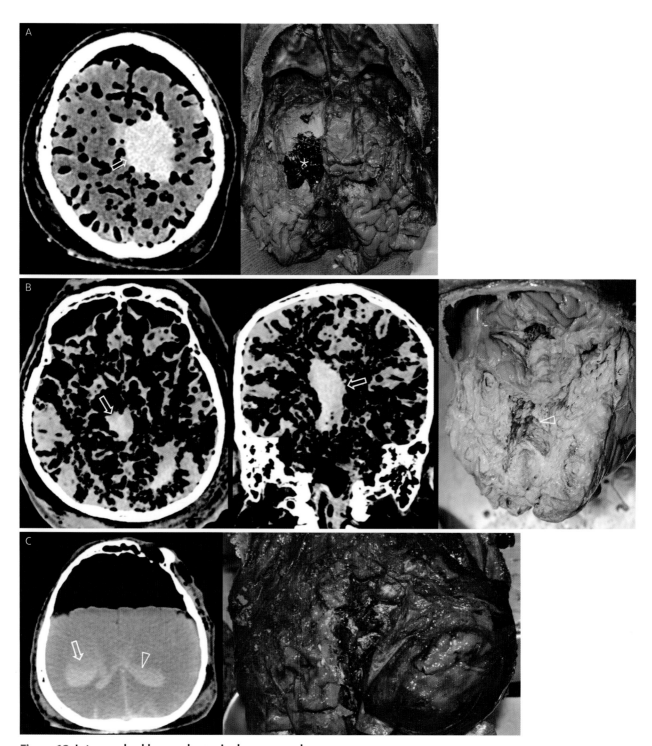

Figure 12. Intracerebral hemorrhages in decomposed cases.

(A) Axial CT image and autopsy photograph show focal high-density hemorrhage in the left basal ganglia (arrows in left, * in right). (B) Axial (left) and coronal (middle) CT images show focal hemorrhage in the right paraventricular area (arrows in left and middle), a deep region of the brain. Autopsy photograph shows focal hemorrhage (arrowhead in right), but precise localization of the hemorrhage is not possible. (C) Axial CT image shows right paraventricular (arrow) and intraventricular hemorrhages (arrowhead), but the specimen photograph depicts reddish discoloration of partially liquefied brain tissue, which interferes with identification and localization of hemorrhage in the brain during autopsy.

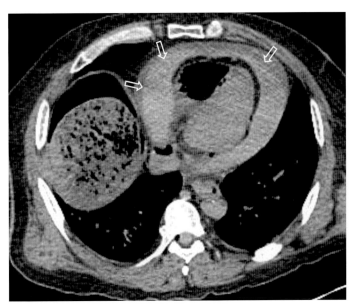

Figure 13. A case of hemopericardium in a male found decomposed.
Axial postmortem CT image shows a double layer of hyperdense inner ring (arrows) and hypodense outer ring (i.e., the hyperdense armored heart sign), indicative of heartbeat during intrapericardial bleeding. This finding is strong evidence of cardiac tamponade as a cause of death.

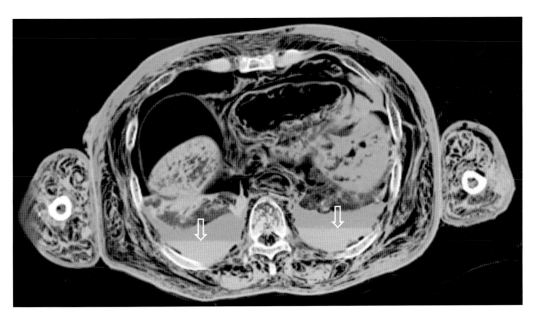

Figure 14. Sedimentation of putrefaction fluid.
Axial CT image shows segmented putrefaction fluid in both pleural cavities with an upper hypodense layer and a lower hyperdense fluid layer (arrows), mimicking blood sedimentation. In this severely decomposed corpse, the upper layer exhibits negative HU values attributable to the presence of fatty contents in the putrefaction fluid, and the lower layer shows HU values that were similar to those of blood from fresh corpses. Therefore, care is needed when CT density is used for the differentiation of body fluid because putrefaction fluid, particularly in a non-sedimented form, can mimic various body fluids (e.g., serous fluid and blood). See Int J Legal Med. 2014; 128:795–802.

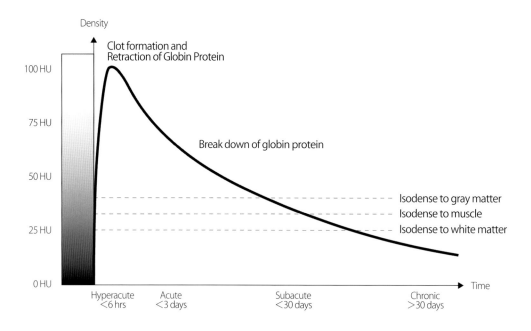

Figure 15. Evolution of antemortem hemorrhage CT density over time.

tion of the clot and resulting in residual areas of tissue loss and parenchymal scarring (**Fig. 15**).[9-11]

In clinical CT imaging, hemorrhage density reaches its maximum within a few hours after the onset of bleeding through clot formation and retraction. If the patient survives beyond this acute phase, the hemorrhage density decreases gradually and becomes hypodense (similar to water) over a few weeks to months. In contrast, the ICH density on PMCT provides a static framework at the time of death in dead bodies, especially with respect to decomposed corpses.[12] This observation indicates that the normal physiological evolution of hemoglobin may cease at the time of death, suggesting that the appearance of hemorrhage on PMCT can be used as a record to de-

termine the age of hemorrhagic blood before death, but is inadequate for estimating the time interval between death and CT examination. Similar to clinical CT, the high density of an acute hematoma can be easily identified on PMCT (including in highly decomposed bodies) and guide autopsy dissection. Although not yet fully understood and systematically investigated, the postmortem cessation of hemorrhage alteration may be useful for reconstructing the perimortem condition of cases with ICH, thereby allowing estimation of the age of hemorrhagic blood at the time of death.[10]

References

1   Levy A, Harcke T. Postmortem Changes and Decomposition. Essentials of Forensic Imaging: A Text-Atlas 1st ed. Boca Raton: CRC Press; 2010. p. 31-52.

2   Knight B, Saukko PJ. Knight's forensic pathology. 3rd ed. Boca Raton, FL: CRC Press; 2004.

3   DiMaio D, DiMaio VJM. Time of Death. Forensic Pathology. 2nd ed. Boca Raten, FL: CRC Press; 2001. p. 21-42.

4   Jason Payne-James J, Busuttil A, Smock W. Forensic Medicine: Clinical and Pathological Aspects. 1st ed. Greenwich Medical Media; 2002.

5   Mann RW, Bass WM, Meadows L. Time since death and decomposition of the human body: variables and observations in case and experimental field studies. Journal of forensic sciences. 1990;35(1):103-11.

6   Shiotani S, Kohno M, Ohashi N, Yamazaki K, Itai Y. Postmortem intravascular high-density fluid level (hypostasis): CT findings. Journal of computer assisted tomography. 2002;26(6):892-3. doi: 10.1097/00004728-200211000-00006.

7   Laczniak AN, Sato Y, Nashelsky M. Postmortem gastric perforation (gastromalacia) mimicking abusive injury in sudden unexplained infant death. Pediatric radiology. 2011;41(12):1595-7. doi: 10.1007/s00247-011-2061-z.

8   Egger C, Bize P, Vaucher P, Mosimann P, Schneider B, Dominguez A, et al. Distribution of artifactual gas on post-mortem multidetector computed tomography (MDCT). International journal of legal medicine. 2012;126(1):3-12. doi: 10.1007/s00414-010-0542-5.

9   Polacco M, Sedati P, Arena V, Pascali VL, Zobel BB, Oliva A, et al. Visualization of myocardial infarction by post-mortem single-organ coronary computed tomography: a feasibility study. International journal of legal medicine. 2015;129(3):517-24. doi: 10.1007/s00414-014-1085-y.

10 Parizel PM, Makkat S, Van Miert E, Van Goethem JW, van den Hauwe L, De Schepper AM. Intracranial hemorrhage: principles of CT and MRI interpretation. European radiology. 2001;11(9):1770-83. doi: 10.1007/s003300000800.

11 Kamalian S, Lev MH, Gupta R. Computed tomography imaging and angiography - principles. Handbook of clinical neurology. 2016; 135:3-20. doi: 10.1016/b978-0-444-53485-9.00001-5.

12 Ruder TD, Zech W, harcke GM, Ross S, Ampanozi G, Thali MJ, et al. Still frame from the hour of death: Acute intracerebral hemorrhage on post-mortem computed tomography in a decomposed corpse. J Forensic Radiol Imag. 2013;1(2):73-6. doi: 10.1016/j.jofri. 2013. 03.042.

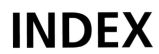

INDEX

A

Agony 155

Air embolism 53, 54, 57, 59, 60, 65, 143, 164

Artifacts
MR artifact 5
Motion induced 15, 106
Streak 16
Histological 19
Perimortem medical intervention 152
Postmortem clot 155
Contrast leakage by autolysis 156
Extravascular contrast diffusion 157
Blood clumping 157
Contrast gravity 159

Animal predation 162

Aorta
Aneurysm
abdominal 4, 132
ascending 105, 106
Dissection 107
Diameter 105
Rupture
ascending 105, 107
isthmus 43, 44
abdominal 4, 131, 132
Vegetation 97

Asphyxia
Chocking 117
food 118
benign neoplasm 120
malignant neoplasm 119
Definition 117
Drowning 85, 86
fresh water 87, 88
salt water 89, 90, 91
Strangulation
definition 80
manual 80, 81, 83
ligature 80, 81, 83
Hanging 80-83

Autopsy findings
Nontraumatic cases
aortic dissection
aortic aneurysm 4, 105, 132
aortic rupture 105, 132
aortic vegetation 97
coronary artery obstruction 98, 99
coronary artery dissection 100
myocardial infarction 101
myocardial rupture 101
hemopericardium 101, 153
intracerebral hemorrhage 109
intracranial hemorrhage in decomposed brain 114, 171, 172
brain stem hemorrhage 111, 112
tumors of neck 119, 120
aspiration of blood into airway 124
bronchopulmonary dysplasia 125
midgut volvulus 134
bowel perforation 135
Trauma-related death
hygroma 36
skull fracture 33, 38
surgical blade injury to skull 142
epidural hemorrhage 38
subdural hemorrhage 36, 38
vertebral artery tear 40, 41
vertebral body fracture 48
burnt body injury 48, 51
spinal cord hemorrhage 51
cardiopulmonary resuscitation-related injuries 154
penetrating injury of skull 61
thyroid cartilage fracture 81
hyoid bone fracture 82

B

Blast injury
Blast wave 72, 73
Shock wave 72-74
Blast wind 72, 73
Negative atmospheric pressure 73
Classification 73, 75
landmine explosion 74, 76
role of CT 75, 77